Carole Lewis

BEST-SELLING AUTHOR OF *THE DIVINE DIET*

STOP IT!

Regal

From Gospel Light
Ventura, California, U.S.A.

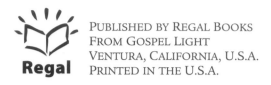

PUBLISHED BY REGAL BOOKS
FROM GOSPEL LIGHT
VENTURA, CALIFORNIA, U.S.A.
PRINTED IN THE U.S.A.

Regal Books is a ministry of Gospel Light, a Christian publisher dedicated to serving the local church. We believe God's vision for Gospel Light is to provide church leaders with biblical, user-friendly materials that will help them evangelize, disciple and minister to children, youth and families.

It is our prayer that this Regal book will help you discover biblical truth for your own life and help you meet the needs of others. May God richly bless you.

For a free catalog of resources from Regal Books/Gospel Light, please call your Christian supplier or contact us at 1-800-4-GOSPEL *or* www.regalbooks.com.

Library of Congress Cataloging-in-Publication Data
Lewis, Carole, 1942-
    Stop it! / Carole Lewis.
        p. cm.
    ISBN 0-8307-3839-8 (hard cover)
    1. Self-control—Religious aspects—Christianity. I. Title.

BV4647.S39L49 2005
248.4—dc22   2005027269

1   2   3   4   5   6   7   8   9   10   /   10   09   08   07   06   05

Rights for publishing this book in other languages are contracted by Gospel Light Worldwide, the international nonprofit ministry of Gospel Light. For additional information, visit www.gospellightworldwide.org; write to Gospel Light Worldwide, P.O. Box 3875, Ventura, CA 93006; or send an e-mail to info@gospellightworldwide.org.

Contents

Introduction 5

Chapter 1 7
The Jolt That Moves Us
It's a small phrase, but it can change our lives.

Part 1: HEART

Chapter 2 21
Stop Losing; Start Choosing
When the fight to feel good moves us toward temptation, it's time to enlist a stronger strategy.

Chapter 3 33
Stop Blaming; Start Answering
When someone else is always at fault, that's just too convenient to be true.

Chapter 4 45
Stop Surviving; Start Thriving
Life is either a problem to be solved or a journey to be enjoyed—the choice is ours.

Part 2: SOUL

Chapter 5 57
Stop Wondering; Start Believing
God is good, and He cares for us. So why do we doubt it?

Chapter 6 67
Stop Worrying; Start Trusting
Because we're in God's hands, we have nothing to worry about—ever!

Chapter 7 77
Stop Wavering; Start Obeying
If we say that we love God, we need to obey Him.

Part 3: MIND

Chapter 8 89
Stop Indulging; Start Considering

We can give in to every urge, or we can focus on the consequences. One way leads to hurt, the other way to health.

Chapter 9 101
Stop Absorbing; Start Discerning

Embracing everything that comes our way is a sure track to a cluttered mind. Filtering life through God's Word produces a clear view of reality.

Chapter 10 111
Stop Controlling; Start Empowering

Trying to dictate what happens in our world only wears us out. Only when we allow people to make choices and live with the consequences are we on the road to health.

Part 4: STRENGTH

Chapter 11 123
Stop Relapsing; Start Resisting

Once we get going on the right path, it's easy to fall back into harmful habits. We must make plans to guard our life.

Chapter 12 135
Stop Retreating; Start Running

Stopping a destructive habit and replacing it with a healthy one is the first big step. But we can't leave it at that. Sustaining the new habit is all-important if we truly want to succeed.

Chapter 13 145
Stop Deviating; Start Tracking

Make a plan and stick to it. It's that simple.

Chapter 14 155
Staying Stopped; Staying Started

Final thoughts for the road ahead.

Introduction

Comedian Bob Newhart once played a psychologist with a unique knack for solving people's problems.

In one sketch, a woman came to him with a very troubled state of mind and told him she had a fear of being locked inside a box.

Bob asked her if she had ever been locked in a box. "No," she replied.

Bob then said, "If you've never been locked in a box, then you aren't going to be locked in a box. STOP IT!"

When the woman told Bob that she made herself throw up after she ate, he said, "Are you bulimic?" When she answered yes, he responded, "That's crazy. Why would you do that? STOP IT!"

"Well," the woman said, "I also have this habit of washing my hands all the time."

"Oh, that's fine," Bob responded, "There's a lot of germs out there; I do that too."

!

I started thinking about that sketch last holiday season. I was at my daughter's home on Christmas Eve and again on Christmas day and found myself eating too many sweets. It was a pattern I knew would be harmful to me, but for some reason, I just couldn't say no.

I decided that I would use those two simple words, "stop it," until I could get back on track. The next day, every time I even thought about eating something I shouldn't, I yelled "STOP IT!" My husband, Johnny, and I had a lot of fun with it. After just one day of doing this, I had stopped a destructive eating pattern.

As funny as it may sound, a profound truth exists in Bob Newhart's straightforward advice. Stopping the negative is an absolute prerequisite for experiencing the success we all desire. Once we have *stopped* harmful patterns, we are able to *start* healthy patterns. Replacing the bad with the good has the power to open up a life we might have never dreamed could be possible—a life of purpose, meaning, wholeness and health.

That's what this book is about. With God's help and the right mind-set, you and I can start the process of destroying negative habits and rebuilding positive ones to get on the right track today. The amazing life you desire is well within your grasp.

If that sounds worthwhile to you, I invite you to keep reading.

—Carole

CHAPTER 1

The Jolt That Moves Us

It's a small phrase, but it can change our lives.

All hard work brings a profit, but mere talk leads only to poverty.
PROVERBS 14:23

Have you ever wished that you could
> *stop thinking* certain thoughts,
>> *stop acting* a particular way,
>>> *stop returning* again and again to bad habits

so that you could be a different person than you are now?

You're not alone.

Maybe right now you would have to admit that everything isn't the way it's supposed to be in your life. Sure, there are good moments, but there are also moments—sometimes there are whole seasons—when you just feel sick of yourself. That's when you might have to say, in all honesty, that there are one or two areas of your life that aren't good at all.

And that matters. Those destructive areas affect your whole person—what you tell yourself, what you think and how you act. Maybe one of those "not good" areas in your life is your weight. It's tough for you to even walk up a flight of stairs.

Maybe your situation involves your kids. Whenever you say anything, they just roll their eyes, declaring that their world is cool and yours isn't. Maybe all communication between you and your husband right now is negative or even nonexistent. Whenever the two of you are together, it seems like he just tunes you out.

Regardless of the specific details, the bottom line is the same and is quite apparent in those moments when we're 100 percent honest about what we're going through. In those candid moments, we might whisper,

- I'm a horrible mother (father).
- I'm a dreadful wife (husband).
- I'm not a very good example to others.
- I'm a bad employee.
- I'm an awful leader.

Ouch!

Your situation, however, is not hopeless. You know that a more positive way exists. You can see something better. Deep down you long to be the kind of person you admire. He or she has more patience than you, more joy, more peace or happiness, doesn't quit, doesn't lose his or her temper, never gives up hope. This person's life is characterized by discipline and satisfaction.

But that's not me, you sigh.

And that's the problem.

A Jolting Solution

There is a solution to what you're going through right now, although the answer may not be as gentle as you think it should be. If I were in the same room as you, I'd shout it as loud as I could. I'd shout

STOP IT!!!!!
Just STOP IT!!
STOP IT! and STOP IT! and STOP IT again!!! (Is that
a jolt or what?!)

Perhaps those are not the words you wanted to hear, but
they do represent the simple truth behind solving so much of
the yucky stuff in our lives. Life doesn't just magically happen.
God designed us to play a part in the way we change. We've got
to stop doing certain negative things before we can start doing
the positive things that are going to help us. So, *STOP IT!*

Stopping destructive thoughts and actions has the power to
open up a life you think could never be possible. This good life,
filled with meaning and purpose, is well within your grasp. To
experience it, however, you must stop the bad on the way to starting the good.

This new way of thinking and acting involves two key components. The first component is *our will*. We have to firmly
decide to take a plan of action, however small or large it may be,
and then do it. The second component is that we have to depend
on *the changing power of the Holy Spirit* in our lives. God is ultimately the One who creates lasting, good change in our hearts
and lives. Yes, God changes us, but we must play a role too.
Neither component can be ignored. We've got to want to change
and then take steps in that direction. With God's power, we will
accomplish what we want to change.

Can a changed life come about as simply as choosing to
stop doing something and praying for God's help in the
process? Absolutely. As we learn to "catch" our destructive
thoughts when they come to mind, we can take captive those
thoughts to make them obedient to Christ (see 2 Cor. 10:5).
When we adjust destructive thoughts before they take root in
our minds and hearts, we can change the destructive behaviors

that result from those thoughts.

For example, imagine an afternoon when you're feeling down for whatever reason. You want to do something that makes you feel better. What are your thoughts? If you think you can never exercise, then you never will. If you think that overeating is the solution, it always will be. But just before you devour that box of doughnuts, you can stop the thought that has just lied to you and take it captive.

Just STOP IT!!! you say.

STOP IT! STOP IT! STOP IT!!!!!

And so you walk away from the donuts. Why? Because eating an entire box of donuts as a way to feel better is always a destructive behavior. It will never give you the lasting peace, satisfaction or health you desire. So you adjust that thought. You know that the way to feel better is to take a walk or do something else that will be good for you and will take your mind off the donuts. What do you do? You commit. You lace up your walking shoes and let your new actions reflect your new thoughts.

Sounds easy, doesn't it—almost too easy. It's not. But it works. Our commitment plus God's help can yield some incredible changes in our lives. That's the foundation for what this book is about.

It's also true that wanting lasting change and actually achieving it are not as simple as we may think. The body wants to do what the body wants to do. Seldom do we wake up in the morning and think: *Goody, goody—I get to exercise today,* or *Yippee, every bite I eat today will be good for me.* The apostle Paul describes this struggle in 1 Corinthians 9:27: "I beat my body and make it my slave." In the same passage, Paul compares his life to an athlete who goes into strict training. He's running a race to get a prize. He runs with purpose, he says; he's not just running aimlessly.

So what's our purpose? What's the race we need to run?

Our race is to fulfill our life's calling to be healthy, whole people who live lives of victory and purpose. Our race is to take a sincere look at our lives and to be able to say with honesty, humility and confidence

- I'm a good mother (father).
- I'm a caring and loving wife (husband).
- I'm an example of progress and growth to others.
- I'm a competent employee.
- I am the leader God wants me to be.

The mind-set that Paul describes can be ours, regardless of our level of athletic ability. What sort of jogger we may or may not be is not the point. The point is that we must want to change. The Lord knows that without a healthy life, we're going to be miserable inside and out. To live a healthy life, we must be committed to the process the same way an athlete commits to a race.

Are you ready for that commitment? Sometimes change is scary, even if it's good change. Typically, when we're facing change, we surround ourselves with our habits as a means of protecting or soothing ourselves. When we start to change, suddenly those old protective devices aren't there anymore. Sometimes even our identity is wrapped up in our bad habits. We've always been known as "the jolly fat person" or "the person who wasn't able to chaperone her teenager's trip because she couldn't fit in a plane seat." We may fear that when we change—even when we change for the better—we won't know who we are anymore or that we'll be asked to do things we've never done before.

And that might happen. Life isn't as predictable as we want it to be. But our decisions in this area come back to our knowledge and confidence of God as good. What does the Bible tell us about our Lord? It says that God has good plans for us, and He wants to rescue us from the wretched situations of our lives.

Romans 8:28 tells us that He works all things out for good. Jeremiah 29:11 reminds us that God's plans are to prosper and not to harm us. But He's got to have our cooperation, too. God isn't in the business of twisting our arms, forcing us to do something we don't want to do. We must be open to the Lord and willing to change for the better.

We can do this! A better way of living is well within our grasp. Our call today is to stop doing certain negative things before we can start doing the positive things that are going to help us. We must stop the bad on the way to starting the good.

Your "Stop It" Plan Begins Here

As this book unfolds, you will begin to recognize that you want a better way of living. You'll recognize that you can choose this path—*you can choose to change*. You'll find that as you take steps to change destructive behaviors in your life, harmful habits can indeed be stopped. And you'll begin to replace harmful habits with positive habits that enrich your life and provide health, purpose and vitality.

One of the key themes in this book is *maintenance*. Your dictionary would define "maintenance" as keeping something in an existing state. Have you ever noticed that we can maintain both bad and good habits? We can either maintain a decision to eat a tub of ice cream every time we feel bad or, when we're feeling the same way, we can maintain a decision to phone a friend, walk the dog or read a good book.

Maintenance is a positive and exciting concept *only if* we are on the right side of the word. To maintain something that no longer works or, for that matter, may have never worked in the first place is ludicrous. Yet this is what many of us do every day. We maintain destructive thoughts and actions that have never worked and will never work, all the while hoping that our destructive patterns will change.

In the pages ahead, we will take a look at some of the broken areas of our lives that we need to *stop* maintaining. Our aim is to change those actions and thoughts and replace them with maintenance on the positive side of things. Replacing bad habits with good habits is just the beginning. One of our goals will be to build sustainable positive habits that we can enjoy for the rest of our lives. Once we build positive thoughts and actions, we will want to nurture and practice them for the rest of our days.

Since we humans are complex beings, we will also take a look at every area of our lives using the fourfold approach to living found in Jesus' words in Mark 12:30: "Love the Lord your God with all your *heart* and with all your *soul* and with all your *mind* and with all your *strength*" (emphasis added). We'll examine each of these areas of life: Heart (the emotional aspect), Soul (the spiritual aspect), Mind (the mental aspect) and Strength (the physical aspect). Think of yourself as a four-sided person. All four sides need to be balanced to keep things in place.

God is a good God, and when we're tempted to follow the path of our bad habits, He always gives us a way of escape. First Corinthians 10.13 shows us this powerful promise: "God is faithful; he will not let you be tempted beyond what you can bear. But when you are tempted, he will also provide a way out so that you can stand up under it."

I will say it again: It is possible to change a negative behavior, but to do so, God needs our cooperation. That's something I know only too well.

My Lifelong Battle

Have you ever noticed that God often creates ministries for us in the areas in which we struggle the most? It seems as though God knows that we have to be allowed to experience something first-hand before we're able to speak to people in that area with confidence. Many times God will use the worst possible thing that could happen to us to become our area of ministry.

For example, author and speaker Chuck Colson has a tremendous ministry today with Prison Fellowship, equipping and assisting the Church in its ministry to prisoners, ex-prisoners and their families. Chuck is able to have so much positive influence because he was once incarcerated for his involvement with the Watergate scandal. He knows firsthand what it's like to be in jail, and because of this, he can effectively and powerfully empathize with those to whom he ministers.

My "jailhouse" is dessert. I've spent a lot of time there—too much time.

It's a habit I'm not proud of, but I want to be honest with you in sharing my struggles in this area. My temptation is not just any dessert: it's specifically *creamy* dessert. I won't go into prolonged descriptions of my craving, but let's just say it's very real. Cheesecake is my favorite dessert by far. It doesn't even matter what type of cheesecake. Although some are better than others, I haven't met a cheesecake I didn't like.

I wish I could say cheesecake liked me in return.

My weight-loss journey didn't start until my late 30s and early 40s. I had three teenagers by then and it seemed like my metabolism had slowly but definitely gone on strike over the years. I'm not a tall person—about five feet three inches when I stand against a wall—so a fluctuation of 20 pounds will make me jump three dress sizes. And jump I had.

I remember a day back in 1981— I was a year away from turning 40—when a friend's casual comment stopped me cold. We were at a baby shower. My friend had lost 20 pounds—the same amount I needed to lose. When I asked her how she could lose so much and not tell me, she said, "Carole, we're going to be 40 next year. You don't want to be fat and 40, do you?"

Fat and 40. Now that had a ring to it I just couldn't handle. So in March 1981, when my church announced the launch of First Place—a weight-loss program that not only addressed physical health but advocated and taught balance in all areas of life—I joined.

Now that I am national director of First Place, you would think I'd have weight-loss maintenance completely under control. Well, let me just say that it's easy for me to go back to my old ways. All the poor habits I gained in the first 40 years of my life are still familiar to me today. I know the signs, the temptations, the tendencies, the rationalizations—all that goes into eating for all the wrong reasons.

Just last week, I found myself slipping back into an old destructive pattern of mine. My husband, Johnny, has been battling stage-four prostate cancer for eight years now. He's done very well, but some seasons are just harder than others. Lately, he's been having a bout with his gallbladder and was in the hospital for several days following his second gallbladder attack, needing surgery. During that particular time, he had a really rough go of it. We were in California when he had the first attack, and he was also in the middle of a round of chemotherapy. The chemo, combined with the two gallbladder attacks, caused him to lose 30 pounds. He looked frail and peaked. His arm was in bad shape from a drug infiltration and, to top it off, we had not gotten along really well with all of his doctors during this treatment. It was a stressful time—just the kind of time when I tend to get in trouble with my eating

So there I was in the hospital cafeteria on a day when Johnny had experienced a particularly bad day. I desperately wanted something that would make me feel better. That desire, combined with being alone in a place that serves food, is not a good combination. I resisted at first. I had a nice, sensible chicken filet sandwich for lunch. (Victory.) I even passed on the chips. (Victory again.) After I finished the sandwich, that feeling surfaced again—wanting something to eat to make me feel better. Notice that I didn't pray or quote Scripture. The thought had resurfaced and I did nothing to STOP IT.

It was a piece of buttermilk pie that did me in. I had seen it as I went through the cafeteria line.

Such a small piece of pie, I thought.

I ate it, I must say, for all the wrong reasons. Later, in the hospital snack shop, with the taste of buttermilk pie still on my lips, I downed a creamy candy bar in one fell swoop. The slope got more slippery the more I gave in. I never keep any bad food in the house, but on the drive home that night, I found myself searching for fast-food outlets, craving an ice-cream cone. *Pie. Candy bar. Ice-cream cone.* What would be next? This was certainly not practicing maintenance on the positive side of things. Johnny was having a bad day, and I was only eating to make myself feel better. I was turning to food for comfort and solace. I wanted creamy desserts to be my savior, but they would only be my jail unless or until I could say STOP IT! Can you see what a destructive path I had chosen?

I've written eight books now, and anything I've ever written about, I've had to live through first. I know firsthand what it's like to wish that I could

> *stop* thinking certain thoughts,
> > *stop* acting a particular way,
> > > *stop* returning again and again to bad habits

so that I could be a different person.

I know what it's like to need to stop doing certain negative things before I can start doing the positive things that are going to help me. It's a lifelong quest to STOP IT, and I'm with you on this journey. My aim is to go forward. I know it's the best way, and I know it can be done.

Success Is Close; Success Is Here

This is my promise to you: If you want your life to change, it will. As you learn to STOP IT, your new habits will replace the bad ones. Stopping our destructive thoughts and actions has the power to bring us a life filled with meaning and purpose. This good life is well within our grasp, but we must stop the bad on the way to starting the good.

It will take time—so be patient and give yourself permission to fail. But remember, you can do it! You are an overcomer in Christ, and you can say with confidence that God has something better for you than what you're experiencing right now.

I'd like you to do one thing. Take a moment and imagine the possibilities of your life. I want you to stop looking at who you are today and start looking at who you can become. In every one of us, there's a winner. Sometimes the winner is hidden, but we just need to find the key to unlock our potential. For me, the key is plain and simple obedience to Christ. When I ask for help, He gives it to me. Life is made up of one choice after another. Let's choose to make the right choices today.

Will you join me on this path?

Prayer

Dear Lord, I know that my life isn't all it could be right now, but with Your help, I'm willing to start on another path. I commit to Your plan for my life, and Your plan is always good. With Your help, I know I'll succeed. Thank You for always being so good. Amen.

PART 1:

—HEART—

Our emotions are valid, but our feelings can overtake us if we allow them. We especially run into problems when our feelings aren't based in fact. In turn, these feelings can cause us to think and act in ways that are destructive to our lives and to the lives of those around us.

Our life goal is to function optimally so that we can serve God each day. By stopping destructive behaviors, we will start to find healthy ways of dealing with our emotions.

That's what the next three chapters will discuss.

CHAPTER 2

Stop Losing;
Start Choosing

When the fight to feel good moves us
toward temptation,
it's time to enlist a stronger strategy.

---

*God is faithful; he will not let you be tempted beyond what you
can bear. But when you are tempted, he will also provide a
way out so that you can stand up under it.*
1 CORINTHIANS 10:13

Years ago, I realized that I should never go near Baskin-Robbins.

Not every store, mind you, just one specific store on the way
to where I used to work at Long Point Baptist Church in
Houston. It's funny, but I can't even remember what kind of car
I drove back then; but I do remember the names of the streets
where the ice cream store was located: Bingle Road, off Westview
Drive.

Actually (ahem), the store wasn't en route to my work at all.
I just convinced myself that it was.

That was the problem.

I had my strategy carefully mapped out. Since all three of
our kids went to school on the same campus as the church, we

would drive in together. I was seldom tempted to stop at Baskin-Robbins when the kids were with me, because of the expense of four ice-cream cones. But once the kids were safely in their classes and I was at work, it seemed there was always some reason for me to go out by myself during the day: office supplies, a trip to the post office—that sort of thing. And on the way back, well, if I stayed on Westview Drive, it was a straight shot back to the church.

But the siren call to turn left on Bingle always beckoned.

I made all sorts of rationalizations: *I won't actually stop for ice cream today*; *I'll just drive down Bingle Road because I enjoy the view.* Who was I kidding? There was only one reason I turned left on Bingle. I knew exactly where I was going and what I would do once I got there. It was Pralines and Cream I was after. I would always get a cone (can't eat ice cream in a dish when you drive). This was my time—my treat—just a little afternoon pick-me-up. The route down Bingle Road was a longer route back to the church—many more stoplights than going straight on Westview—but all those stops before I got back to the office gave me the perfect opportunity to savor the cone.

Day after day, I lost my battle for a healthy lifestyle by giving in to my familiar craving. Stopping for ice cream had nothing to do with being hungry. It was emotional eating through and through. Food, especially sweets, brings me back to the emotions of the good childhood I experienced. Whenever I eat ice cream, it's like I'm a little kid again, and Mom has baked a cake on a Saturday afternoon. Warm emotions and food go hand in hand in my life. Food equals pleasure, safety, security, sanctuary. After eating ice cream, I'd go back to the office happy as a clam.

Why did I need a pick-me-up? It wasn't as if my life was horrible back then at all—no, the craving was much more subtle than that. I would give in to my temptation because it just scratched an itch. I liked to please myself. I wanted to feel good, and the power of my craving offered me a temptation I could not resist. Yet the fact was, every time I made a left turn onto Bingle Road, I lost.

If I was ever going to win the war to

> *stop* thinking certain thoughts,
>> *stop* acting a particular way,
>>> *stop* returning again and again to bad habits

so that I could be a different person, I needed to enlist a stronger strategy.

The Battle for Our Emotions

What is your Bingle Road? What is the specific something that makes you lose the battle toward healthy living? Bingle Road takes you to a place you shouldn't go. We all have some sort of craving that moves us toward temptation. Wanting to feel good, which is a natural desire, isn't the problem. The problem is when we turn to something that isn't healthy for us in order to feel good—particularly if it seems as though we're powerless over the craving.

For example, my mother's Bingle Road was probably a bag of jellybeans at the grocery store checkout counter. Whenever she wheeled her cart to the cashier, there they were. And she always bought them. Jellybeans were her emotional reward for the day. She ate them because they made her feel good. And when she ate jellybeans, she lost.

Our cravings don't have to be about food. For some people, it's alcohol. After a long day at work or home, the only thing that makes some people feel better is a couple glasses of red wine before bed. When they're honest, they realize a dependency has taken place; if they don't have the wine, they can't sleep. That's losing the battle in the fight to feel good.

For others, the siren call is work. Our lives always contain some sort of chaos, and sometimes it seems as though the only way to avoid dealing with negative feelings is to throw ourselves into our jobs. People can also use church activities this way. The logic is that because thinking and feeling can be painful, we won't have time to think or feel if we stay busy. But keeping busy for the sake of masking our true emotions means that we're lying to ourselves. And we lose.

Studies show that for many men today (for some women, too), their Bingle Road is pornography. Perhaps a man feels that he's not getting the respect he deserves, or that his spouse is too busy or too critical—whatever the excuse, pornography seems to be the answer, the instant remedy for how he feels. But pornography is a lie, just like all Bingle Road experiences.

Years ago, there was a woman at work whose Bingle Road was to complain. It seemed as though every day she'd find 10 things to get frustrated about. She'd walk from office to office spilling her annoyances on everyone she met. Her life was habitually characterized by negativity, and her method of dealing with her feelings was to spew her complaints on her coworkers. It was pure emotional vomit. Oh, I loved this woman, but what a downer she could be! Her emotions ruled her. Her constant venting was hard on her too; she developed a reputation as a grumbler and complainer. Eventually, she quit and moved on, but I doubt her attitude changed, and I wonder how long she lasted at her next job.

What is your Bingle Road? What is that one area that tempts you again and again? What is the one thing that once you head down its road, you know you're in a place you shouldn't be?

Take a few moments to write some thoughts in a journal or in the space on the next page. Be as specific as you can. Write down the circumstances, the times, the places, people, events and locations that move you toward temptation.

My Bingle Road is _____.

It tends to happen at the following place(s) _____
_____

at the following time(s) _____

when these types of things are happening in my life: _____
_____.

When I give in to my Bingle Road, I initially feel _____
_____.

But afterward, I usually feel _____
_____.

The Bible tells us that our Bingle Roads are part of being human. First Corinthians 10:13 reads: "No temptation has seized [us] except what is common to man." Being tempted is part of life, but we don't have to give in to temptation.

There's a powerful promise in this verse as well: "God is faithful; he will not let you be tempted beyond what you can bear. But when you are tempted, he will also provide a way out so that you can stand up under it."

There is a way to stop losing. But we have to choose it.

The Shout That Provides a Way Out

What's the solution? I bet you know what I'm going to say.

STOP IT!

Just STOP IT!

STOP IT! and STOP IT!! and STOP IT again!!!!

Until we can learn to shout STOP IT! at the crossroads of

choosing harmful experiences, we will forever take that left turn off of Westview Drive and head down Bingle road to what destroys us.

Think about it: Your Bingle Roads are vicious. They hurt you. They never bring the lasting joy and lasting satisfaction you hope they will. They affect who you are, what you tell yourself, what you think and how you act. Unless you say STOP IT! before these experiences start, you will be doomed to repeat your damaging behaviors.

Your situations are never hopeless. Stopping your destructive thoughts and actions has the power to open up a life you never dreamed possible—a life filled with meaning and purpose. This good life is well within your grasp. But you must stop the bad on the way to starting the good. You've got to stop losing—in this case, losing the battle in the fight for your emotions. You stop losing by starting to choose—in this case starting to make choices that keep you heading in the right direction. It may take time. You need to be patient with yourself and give yourself permission to fail. But you can do it. You are an overcomer in Christ, and you can say with confidence that God has something better for you than your Bingle Road.

I'd like to suggest a strong strategy that will help you stop losing and start choosing. This strategy will head you in the right direction. Think of this as a map that gives you power to drive toward a better, healthier, sustainable lifestyle.

Recognize the Wrong Road
Sometimes it's hard to even know that you have a problem, isn't it? You can sail along in life, simply going through the same routines every day. But maybe there's a nagging ache in the pit of your stomach. Or maybe it's just a tiny voice in the back of your head. The problem may not be obvious at first, but if you listen, you'll know something is not the way it's supposed to be.

Sometimes you're hesitant to call a problem a problem or to admit you have a problem in the first place. But a problem is a problem if something interferes with your life. Is something hindering your marriage? Your relationship with your kids? Your time at work? Your relationships in your church community?

The first step in this strategy is to recognize that a wrong road exists. Who was I fooling when I kept turning left from Westview onto Bingle Road on the way to Baskin-Robbins? For me, that road led to one place and one place only. I needed to recognize this fact in my life. I was eating emotionally, and it was harming me. I needed to see this fact and recognize it for what it was.

What truth do you need to recognize? What's out of whack right now in your life?

Name the Wrong Road

Once a problem has been recognized, you need to name it. Some people skip this step, but I believe it's very important. You need to say your problem out loud or write it down. When you do this, you begin to understand and can list the specifics of the problem—it helps to identify definite points that tempt you in the battle to stop losing and start choosing.

For example, perhaps your problem is with overeating. It's great to recognize the problem, but it's not enough to leave it at that. Just saying that you have a problem with "food" is too generic. When you name something, you give it corners—your problem becomes concrete and tangible. I would say my problem's name was "eating Pralines and Cream ice cream every time I leave the office alone to run an errand." The name you give your problem doesn't have to be that long, but the point is to give it an identity. Naming the problem helps you see the truth of the situation and helps you understand the specifics of how you interact with that problem. Once you name a problem, it's not as overwhelming. You're not fighting some sort of vague theory, situation or philosophy anymore. Naming a problem helps break it down to size.

Just for the sake of example, let's say you recognize that you have a problem with pornography. Identifying the problem is the first step. But how do you handle the problem? The topic is too broad—too unclear. You must give that wrong road a name. What might be the specifics of your situation if the problem was pornography? Perhaps its name would be "Hotel Room." Your work involves travel, and every time you go to a hotel alone, you're tempted to purchase in-room adult entertainment. Now you've just clarified the specifics of your problem. That's good. Giving it a name helps you see the problem more plainly and helps you stop losing and start choosing.

Lay the Wrong Road on Christ

Our commitment plus God's help can yield some incredible changes in our lives. That's the foundation for what this book is about. Once we admit that we have a problem, and give it a name, we need to lay that problem at the foot of the Cross. This simply means that we ask for God's help in this area. We commit the problem to Him in prayer and ask for His power to change our lives.

God has only good plans for us, and He has a way of doing things that are ultimately for our best. Our prayer can be something as simple as:

Dear Lord, You know I've got a problem with

_____.

Please help me. I cannot overcome this area by myself.
It is too big.
I commit this area to You.
With Your help, I'll succeed.
Amen.

In John 6:35, Jesus tells us that He alone has the power to ultimately satisfy our lives. "I am the bread of life. He who comes to me will never go hungry, and he who believes in me will never be thirsty." Whenever we crave something, what we are really longing for is a type of satisfaction that only Jesus Christ can bring.

Galatians 5:16 tells us to live by the Spirit. When we do, we "will not gratify the desires of the sinful nature." What our sinful natures desire is what harms us. But prayer can enable us to live by the Spirit's power if we truly know Jesus as our Lord and Savior. When we lay our problems at the foot of the Cross, we will have the power to stop losing and start choosing.

Another great Scripture passage in this area is Philippians 4:6-7: "Do not be anxious about anything, but in everything, by prayer and petition, with thanksgiving, present your requests to God. And the peace of God, which transcends all understanding, will guard your hearts and your minds in Christ Jesus."

When we purposely cast our anxiety on the Lord, we have the wonderful promise found in that verse—that Christ will provide safety and security for our hearts and our minds. That's certainly a comfort. Christ cares for us, and He will give us the strength we need.

Choose to Drive on the Right Road

The final step in this strategy is our responsibility. When we find ourselves at a crossroads moment, we must shout STOP IT! or else we will turn down the wrong path. We have to stop the behavior that leads us to destruction. Our feelings follow our actions. So over time, choosing to take the healthy path *will* become easier.

Don't worry! When you stop old harmful behaviors, you may become anxious and uneasy at first—you've been used to the same patterns for so long. But you must stop losing the battle that leads you down destructive paths, and start choosing healthy paths.

Choosing the right path is a learned behavior. You make it consciously. At this point you have named your problem area. Now you need to avoid it. How do you avoid it? You choose to. It's that simple.

For example, do you go from office to office at work, complaining to everyone you meet? STOP IT! Make a conscious decision that the next time you feel frustrated, you won't vent to your colleagues about it. Stop losing. Start choosing. What do you choose in this case? You choose to express your frustrations in a healthy manner. Maybe that means writing them down in a journal. Maybe it means taking a walk around the building.

Do you buy a candy bar every time you get to the checkout counter? STOP IT! Make a conscious decision to remind yourself every time you go shopping that you won't achieve an emotional pick-me-up with candy. Stop losing and start choosing. What will you choose? Perhaps in this case, you'll eat a healthy snack, such as a banana or an orange. Perhaps it will mean going shopping at a time of the day when you won't feel as vulnerable. Stop losing and start choosing.

The Strong Strategy

We were created by God to have emotions, and it's okay to experience them. But our emotions will cripple us if we let them. If our emotions are moving us toward temptation, we need to enlist a stronger strategy. That strategy is to stop losing and start choosing.

As you become willing to take an honest look at every aspect of your life, God will come in if you ask Him and help you stop the things that are keeping you from being and doing all that He desires. Your part is to stop the destruction. God's part is to start the rebuilding.

You can do this. The power is within your grasp to move to a healthy life you never dreamed imaginable. But you've got to want to change, and you've got to take steps in that direction.

With God's help, you will.

Stop Blaming;
Start Answering

When someone else is always at fault, that's just
too convenient to be true.

See . . . that no bitter root grows up.
HEBREWS 12:15

I have a friend who I will call Cindy. She blamed her husband for almost everything that went wrong in the first 25 years of their 45-year marriage. Few things were ever Cindy's fault. Fault usually lay with her husband—I'll call him Chuck. It wasn't that Cindy thought she was blameless, but she reasoned that if the Lord would just change Chuck, it would make her happy.

They married young—both still in college—and moved in with his parents. Money was tight, and kids came along soon. Chuck worked in law enforcement, then corporate security. The couple soon discovered their personalities were complete opposites: Chuck was very vocal and had a quick temper that spilled over at the slightest thing; Cindy was quiet and reserved—she would never argue; she would just cry.

They had challenges in their marriage, but who doesn't?

When they moved into an apartment building, Cindy was hired as the leasing agent, which meant free rent. When the manager was fired, that position came up, and Chuck made Cindy apply for the job. It meant a bigger salary and a free townhouse instead of an apartment. But Cindy didn't want to be manager. She was definitely a behind-the-scenes type of gal. Chuck convinced her to apply. Cindy got the job and hated it. (How could she have known that the Lord was preparing her to manage a large office in her distant future?) Secretly, silently, she blamed Chuck for how miserable she was. And Cindy let her bitterness fester.

Or at least she tried to be silent. She used to read the Bible after dinner while sitting next to Chuck on the couch. As she read, she would say, "Uh huh," every time she read a passage she thought applied to Chuck's life. She did this in a playful way, and it didn't upset Chuck. But he wasn't dumb either. He'd laugh and say, "So you found something about me." Chuck knew that every joke contains an element of truth, and he knew that Cindy was hoping he would read the Bible for himself and that it would change him.

Cindy shared with me a journal entry about how she felt back then. She wrote:

> *Lord, You know my husband needs changing. He has a bad temper; he needs to be the spiritual leader of our family, not me! I read my Bible, go to church and pray. My life would be just fine if you would only change him. It's his fault that I am miserable and unhappy.*

Do you see the blame problem? Cindy was refusing to own the responsibility to communicate her feelings, set some boundaries and create her own happiness.

But the Holy Spirit was at work in Cindy's life.

Somewhere in the midst of meditating on the situation, very gently, the Holy Spirit whispered in Cindy's ear, "There are some things in *your* life that need to be changed. Your heart is dirty with bitterness, unforgiveness, resentment and a stubborn will."

Cindy said she was stunned, but instantly she knew it was the truth.

Why, Lord?!

Have you ever met someone whose life is characterized by blame? Maybe they don't literally point a finger at someone, but the responsibility for their actions always lies with someone else.

When it comes to overeating, people in these situations make statements such as:

- My kids drove me crazy today; I needed an ice-cream sundae.
- My husband brought home a bag of donuts after work. I couldn't say no.
- I was at my coworker's birthday lunch. I had to have a big piece of birthday cake. It was her birthday—what was I supposed to do?

No matter what has gone wrong, it's always someone else's fault. It's the kids, the husband or the coworker who's to blame. Blaming others is a very convenient way of dealing with life. It's so much easier to blame than it is to take responsibility.

We've all heard people say things such as:

- It's my mother's fault that I drink so much. She drank all her life, so I drink, too. It's my way of coping—it's in my genes.
- My husband is so stingy. I go shopping all the time because I know it makes him mad. If he wasn't so rigid, I know I wouldn't spend as much money as I do.
- I only gamble when my wife has PMS. What a grouch. I've just got to get out of the house when she gets like that.
- My coworker Fran is such a whiner. I never have a good day when I'm around her.

Do you notice a pattern here? It's not *my* drinking problem—it's because of my mother's behavior. It's not *my* gambling problem—it's because my spouse is a grouch. And so on.

Blaming others is nothing new. What did Adam and Eve do when God confronted them in the garden? The world's first couple had just eaten from the tree that God commanded them not to touch, but did they 'fess up? The following is my paraphrase of Genesis 3:12-13:

"Uh, Eve made me do it," said Adam.

"Um, it was all the serpent's fault," said Eve.

What a picture of pointing the finger at someone else! We are not alone when it comes to blaming others. It's a convenient practice. But blaming others is ultimately about arrogance. When we blame others, we falsely exonerate ourselves. Blame shifts the burden for wrong actions, thoughts and behaviors onto someone else's shoulders. We're innocent. We're exalted. We wouldn't feel or act this way if they didn't do what they do.

Do you see how prideful this is? Other people may indeed do wrong things. But that is no excuse for not taking responsibility for ourselves. We may live with a husband who is a loafer, work with a colleague who's a back-stabber, raise kids who become rebellious, and mourn for a parent who was never what we hoped he or she would be to us. But that never gives us the excuse to engage in destructive habits. Regardless of the sins of others, we are still responsible for our lives.

When we blame others, we are actually blaming God. We are saying, "Lord, you created this person the way they are. Why, Lord?!" or "Lord, You allowed this situation to exist. You have the power to change things, but You're not doing anything about it. Why, Lord?!"

I have a friend who worked as a youth pastor. Parents of rebellious teens would sometimes approach him with anxiety and fear over their parental situation, but they would also demand that he do something about what was causing their feelings. If nothing changed, it was the youth pastor's fault. My friend worked at a good church where ministries and staff members were in place that would help the teens if they truly wanted to change. But the teens were making poor choices.

Often, the youth pastor would ask these parents if they had prayed about the situation. If the answer was yes, he'd ask, "Why do you think God hasn't changed your son or daughter?" Then the truth would become clearer. It wasn't that God was not willing to help; it was that God was respecting the teenager's choice to rebel. Ultimately, the parents weren't faulting their youth pastor—they were blaming God.

You see, God is a complete Gentleman when it comes to our wills. He gives all people—including teenagers raised in godly homes—the choice to disobey Him. When we're upset at the sins of other people, we're really asking the Lord why He allows sin to exist in the first place. Why does God allow teenagers to be rebellious? Why doesn't God do something about it?! Why, Lord? Why?

And when we blame, we become negative people. Bitterness festers in our lives. And that bitterness hurts us and those around us. The Bible always instructs us to take responsibility for our actions and feelings: "When tempted, no one should say, 'God is tempting me'" (Jas. 1:13).

But how do we do this? How do we own our lives? How do we quit blaming others—and ultimately blaming God?

A Careful Prayer

There is a better way. It is found in two powerful words: STOP IT!

Until we can learn to say STOP IT! we will forever stay mired in the destructive patterns that harm our lives. Blaming others is never the solution. It will never bring the lasting joy and satisfaction we yearn for.

We must stop the bad on the way to starting the good. We can say with confidence that God has something better for us: a life filled with meaning and purpose. But first we have to stop blaming others.

My friend Cindy realized this. She longed for a marriage filled with peace and encouragement. And the Holy Spirit had plans for her life.

Cindy later wrote:

> *I was very sensitive, and through the years my spirit had been wounded with unkind words and the actions of others. Because I did not like conflict, I had unknowingly stored up all these emotions and hurts in my heart. I blamed my misery on my husband.*
>
> *As the Holy Spirit revealed the contents of my heart, I asked Him to remove all the filth from my heart and change me. I asked Him to heal my wounds and restore my marriage.*
>
> *I changed my focus from my husband to me.*

Do you see what Cindy did? She asked the Holy Spirit to change *her* heart. She started taking responsibility for *her* life. And that's the right path to be on!

There is a very important distinction to make at this point. Cindy was not denying her husband's wrongdoings. She wasn't looking at the sin in her husband's life and pretending it wasn't there. She wasn't a doormat who said, "Everything is all my fault." I've seen women do that—they turn the sword on themselves. The truth is nothing like that.

When Cindy took action for her feelings, a positive behavior resulted. She began asking the Lord for His help in the process. She stopped blaming and started taking responsibility.

That's strength and power, and it's true.

God wants us to get better. He wants us to heal. Our situation is never hopeless. It's easy to stay stuck in destructive patterns, but a much better pathway exists. Stopping our destructive thoughts and actions has the power to open a life we never dreamed possible, a life filled with meaning and purpose. And we can start—today.

If you feel that someone else is always the cause of your unhappiness or unfulfillment, let me suggest three practical steps that will get you on the right path.

1. Pray for Insight

The first step is to ask God to show you the contents of your heart. This is not a time to focus on what other people are doing. Others may be wrong, and they may be different, but this isn't about them. It's about you—how you feel and how you act based on those feelings.

Very simply, very directly, you can go to the Lord in prayer. You can ask Him to reveal the truth about your life. You may want to use the words of Psalm 139:23-24 as your prayer: "Search me, O God, and know my heart; test me and know my anxious thoughts. See if there is any offensive way in me, and lead me in the way everlasting."

When your heart is open to Him, God will do the work. In this case, you can trust Him to bring to mind times when you blame others. You can take note of the circumstances around those times. What were you feeling? What were your emotions? Who were you truly mad at? What was your responsibility in the situation?

For example, instead of:

My kids made me so angry, I had to eat a bag of cookies.

Perhaps the truth was:

Truly, my kids were misbehaving. When they act like that, I feel scared that they'll turn out to be horrible people. I feel guilty that maybe I've been a bad parent somewhere along the line. Food gives me comfort—and I go to food instead of taking a more positive approach to the situation. Lord, please help me change this pattern.

2. Take Action

The second step is to stop the destructive behavior of blaming others and to take steps in that direction. How? When you notice that you're in a situation in which you want to blame someone else, you say STOP IT! It's a conscious decision. You may not feel like doing anything other than blame someone. That's natural. You've fallen into the pattern of blaming others for so long that it has become a habit. Pray for willingness and power to stop the destructive pattern.

You can do this. With God's power, you'll make the right choice. Hebrews 12:15 instructs us to "see . . . that no bitter root grows up" in our lives. Not blaming others is a decision you make, even when someone has wronged you. Yet even when you've been wronged, you have many positive options of how to act and feel.

The Bible tells us that we have the choice to forgive, to be thankful in the midst of all circumstances, to put on the full armor of God, to give a gentle answer instead of a harsh one, to "sin not" in our anger, to not let the sun go down on our wrath, to make every effort to live in peace with everyone, to pray for our enemies and do good to those who persecute us, to always be kind to each other, and much more. These are the positive options that are available to us.

3. Release Others

When you begin to focus on your heart—and not on the actions of those around you—paradoxically, the Holy Spirit has much more freedom to work in the lives of others. Blame is a negative emotion, and it makes you and those around you totally miserable. When you stop blaming others and take responsibility for yourself, your life can be characterized by the quiet peace and confidence of knowing that God has an amazing plan for your life. That confidence and peace relaxes people and lays aside the club you might have been holding over them.

What if you're locked in a stalemate of hurt and bitterness with a person? Let's say that person has truly harmed you, and no apology seems forthcoming. Well, someone has to break the stalemate. That's you. Take the responsibility to stop the war. Whatever steps are in your power to take, take them.

My friend Cindy did this. One of the practical steps she took was asking the Holy Spirit to help her remember and write down a list of everyone who had ever hurt her. She started with her childhood and worked forward, putting every instance she could think of on paper. The list grew long. She had an alcoholic father who abandoned the family when Cindy was young. That experience greatly affected Cindy. And because she did not like conflict, she developed a pattern of stuffing her emotions and hurts inside.

One by one, she prayed through each circumstance, asking the Lord to help her forgive the person who had caused her harm, and for the Lord to remove the pain. Some of the people on her list never knew they had hurt Cindy. Some of them were no longer around. But Cindy was not asking anything from these people. She was taking responsibility for her responses to her life's experiences.

We are never called to change other people. That is not our responsibility. Our responsibility is to love Christ and let His love move us to minister as He would have us minister. Changing other people is not in our power, and we frustrate, dishearten and wear ourselves out when we try to make it ours. When we release to the Holy Spirit the responsibility of changing others, we can have true rest. Our work is to point others to the Lord. His work is to change lives.

Welcome to Freedom and Peace

If you are in the habit of blaming others for what goes wrong in your life, then when you stop blaming others and start taking responsibility, just watch what happens. You may not see anything change for a while, but chances are good that things will soon begin to change. You'll see change in yourself first—a freedom and peace that hasn't been there before. And you may see change in others, too. When people are freed from your blame, they have a greater opportunity to become the person the Lord intended.

In Cindy's case, the change was remarkable. She wrote:

As I shifted my focus from my husband to me, miraculously, my husband began to change before my very eyes. He knew nothing of what was happening in my life, because at that time I didn't share what God had shown me. But the amazing thing was that as the Holy Spirit worked in my husband's life, God began using the very things that I had once wanted to change in my husband for purposes I never could have imagined.

God showed me that He makes each of us individually and has a perfect plan uniquely designed for us. God then works through us in different ways to accomplish His plan and purpose on Earth. For example, my husband had always been bold—and at times, his boldness hurt me. But the Lord eventually used his boldness to accomplish mighty things. My husband became a pastor later in life, and his boldness was a positive trait that was evident in prayer and counseling, and in love for other people.

You can do this. You can stop blaming and start taking responsibility. God has a wonderful plan and purpose for you—for each of us. The Lord is waiting for all of us to quit blaming others and to turn our focus on Him. He is the one who "gives generously to all without finding fault" (Jas. 1:5).

Just watch what happens when you're committed to His perfect ways.

CHAPTER 4

Stop Surviving; Start Thriving

Life is either a problem to be solved or
a journey to be enjoyed—the choice is ours.

*Being confident of this, that he who began a good work in you will
carry it on to completion until the day of Christ Jesus.*
PHILIPPIANS 1:6

One of our dear First Place leaders, Stephanie Rhodes, admits
that several years ago, she lived in survival mode. When
Stephanie shares about her life, I can almost feel the blows.

Wham! When Stephanie was in second grade, her best friend
died.

Wham! While still a child, Stephanie discovered her dad was
an alcoholic.

Wham! In junior high, her older brother was diagnosed with
muscular dystrophy.

Wham! In Stephanie's senior year of high school, a favorite
aunt died.

Wham! As a young adult, both her parents became invalids
within years of each other, and Stephanie needed to take care of
them.

Wham! Her brother became confined to a wheelchair and
came to live with her.

Wham! Her sister's marriage fell apart, and the courts became involved in a custody battle with Stephanie's nieces and nephews.

Wham! Her mother was diagnosed with breast cancer and died in Stephanie's arms.

No wonder Stephanie was bruised. One by one, the trials took their toll. Stephanie had no idea what to do with her emotions. Over time, she stuffed her feelings as deeply and tightly as she could.

It's a profound understatement to say that Stephanie needed relief. But during every heartache or disappointment, there was one thing Stephanie turned to. Eating became her way to numb the pain and bring emotional comfort. The destructive habit caught up with her, and major health problems began to develop.

Stephanie wrote:

My whole life was out of order. I became weak in body and spirit, and lost heart, strength and courage. No longer could I tie my own shoes. No longer could I stand more than a minute. A cane became my means of support to walk short distances, and a wheelchair became my mode of transportation if I needed to go very far. Worry had become my lifestyle. I had ceased to hope in the Lord. My desire was not to live, but to die.

Do you know someone in survival mode? When life's events become difficult, it may seem as if the only solution is to stuff the painful emotions so they don't show. But emotions never stay buried for long, despite our greatest efforts to conceal them.

Florence Littauer, one of my greatest mentors in public speaking, compares stuffing our emotions to trying to keep beach balls under water. No matter how hard we push them down, the feelings just pop to the surface! Sometimes they bounce up at strange times and places—like when we're driving a car or are in line at the grocery store. Soon, we realize we don't have control over our lives anymore. Our emotions rule—and they show up as worry, fear, rage, helplessness and hopelessness.

Some years ago I worked with a woman whose emotions would pop to the surface at all the wrong times. One day a group of us were headed out for lunch, although the woman had been invited along, she was nowhere to be found when lunchtime came. So we left instructions for her, saying that we would save her a seat. When she found us, she exploded like a volcano. She spat out the words, "You think you can get rid of me!" What a surprise to us all—and what harm to the woman! Her rage ruled her perception of her circumstances. Her emotions were on the throne.

Another friend, Cheri Lasiter, has cerebral palsy and braces on her legs. Her emotions would surface as fear, which is really anger turned inward. Several years ago Cheri reached a low point in her life when she was unemployed and unable to find something to occupy her time. She would often sit alone in her apartment with the shades down, feeling lonely and full of despair. She had always turned to food for relief, and during this time, would sometimes consume whole cakes.

Cheri was surviving, not thriving. It's easy to fall into the trap.

When our lives become filled with pain, there is a solution—but it's not to stuff our emotions. A more positive way exists. We are overcomers in Christ, and we can say with confidence that God has something better for us than merely surviving. But we have to do something first.

In the Midst of Good Company

I'm going to whisper the solution this time. I'll whisper it, because if you're anything like Stephanie Rhodes, or the woman who exploded over a rearranged lunch date, or Cheri Lasiter sitting alone in her apartment, there's a good chance your life has had its share of harshness. So I want to be gentle yet firm, because there is only one solution to opening up a life of thriving, not surviving.

It's this: Stop it.

Stop it—it's the simple truth behind solving so much of the destructive patterns of our lives. Just stop it. Life does not magically happen. God designed us to play a part in the way we change. And we've got to stop doing certain negative things before we can start doing the positive things that are going to help us.

In this case, if our self-talk is always negative, our lives will follow suit. If we continually tell ourselves that our lives are hopeless, then they will be. If we convince ourselves that we are helpless to change our circumstances, then we will forever stay mired in despondent feelings and the actions that they bring.

So . . . stop it.

Our calling is to be whole people who live with victory and purpose. The Lord knows that without a healthy life, we're going to be miserable inside and out. In order to be healthy, we must want to change. Others have been through the same things we've been through. Their example can offer encouragement and spur us on to excellence.

Check out the story of Moses in Exodus 1–4. Moses had his share of hard knocks. He was effectively orphaned. Though he grew up in opulence, the family he grew up with was never really his. Over time, he developed an anger problem—he even killed an Egyptian and hid his body in the sand. Moses also stuttered. What sort of leader would he ever make? God needed to send him to the backside of a Midian desert for 40 years, schooling Moses in all he needed to know. But when graduation time approached, what did Moses say to God?

Can't do it, Lord. I'll never be the leader You want me to be. Please, can't You send someone else to do it?

Oh, Moses, stop surviving and start thriving.

Abram had his share of problems, too. When a famine came to his land, he fled with his family to Egypt. But he was afraid of the men in the land because his wife was beautiful. So Abram lied about his wife, Sarai, calling her his sister instead. Read the story in Genesis 12:10-20. Abram let fear rule him, and the results were disastrous. You would think he would have learned his lesson, but he did the exact same thing with Abimelech in Genesis 20:1-18.

Abram, just stop it! Stop letting your fear be master of your life. Start immersing yourself in God's promises of care and provision. The Lord will never let you down.

Elijah the prophet is another example of being led astray by emotions. After Elijah raised the dead, slaughtered false prophets, ran up and down Mt. Carmel, and received a death threat from Queen Jezebel, he found himself sitting under a broom tree in the wilderness, praying desperate prayers to God.

"I have had enough, LORD," Elijah says. "Take my life" (1 Kings 19:4).

Can you hear the despondency in this man? Check out the full story in 1 Kings 19. But I love how it ends. The Lord leads Elijah to a cave where a powerful windstorm occurs, but God is not in the wind. Then there's an earthquake, but God's not there either. After the earthquake comes a fire, but still no God. After the fire comes a gentle whisper. When Elijah hears this, he pulls his cloak about him, stands at the mouth of the cave, and prepares to listen to what God has to say.

What does God whisper to Elijah? I'll paraphrase here . . .

Hey, Elijah . . . stop it.

Essentially, God told Elijah that he was not alone and that He still had plans for his life. God told Elijah to stop surviving and start thriving. Notice that God dealt with Elijah's feelings in a gentle way, yet God still dealt with him firmly. Life wasn't hopeless. Elijah wasn't helpless, and God wanted Elijah to know exactly that.

Does the instruction to start thriving seem difficult for us today? James 5:17 says that "Elijah was a man just like us." It doesn't take someone with wonderful self-esteem to be used by God. We don't have to have it all together to begin thriving. It simply takes a yielded life. When we open ourselves to a good God who loves us more than we can imagine, a life we never dreamed possible is waiting.

All for Jesus

When we let the Lord in, miracles happen all the time.

Right now my friend Cheri Lasiter—the same friend with cerebral palsy and braces on her legs—is training to run a 5K race. To date, she's lost over 80 pounds, and the other day, this same woman, who has lived so much of her life in fear, quoted 10 memory verses in front of our First Place group of 30. I am so proud of her! That was an amazing feat when you consider that she used to be petrified of crowds. Cheri stopped surviving and started thriving.

The woman with rage issues? We discovered she had an addiction to painkillers. We helped get her into a rehabilitation program where she kicked the habit and began to work on the real issues that were troubling her life. Today, she is living drug free and enjoying her grandchildren. She stopped surviving and started thriving.

And Stephanie Rhodes? She joined a First Place group and began to immerse herself in Scripture. Even though she has lost more than 125 pounds, her struggles have not ended. She was recently in a horrible car accident and was hospitalized for over a month. But Stephanie realized a strange thing in the midst of this trial.

She wrote:

While firefighters used the Jaws of Life to get me out of my vehicle, for the first time I remember not having fear or worry consume me. I experienced peace that only God can give! During physical rehabilitation in the hospital, God made me aware that He had performed emotional rehabilitation on me as well. Jesus wrapped me in his arms and said: "Draw closer to me, love me and listen to My voice." My prayer now is found in Philippians 1:6—Being confident of this, that He who began a good work in me will carry it on to completion to the day of Christ Jesus our Lord.

That's thriving!

God is a good God who loves us, cares for us, and wants only the best for our lives. Let's look at a few practical ways we can stop surviving and start thriving.

Immersing Our Thoughts in Scripture

Imagine a bathtub at the end of the day. The house is quiet; the kids are asleep. Perhaps candles are lit and soft music is on. Having a good soak in a tub can be one of the most refreshing, soothing, comforting and healing experiences of the day.

The same thing is true with Scripture. Philippians 4:8 instructs us to fill our thoughts with whatever is true, noble, right, pure, lovely and admirable. If we continually fill our thoughts with good things, then we will not have room for fear, anger, rage and anxiety. When our emotions are bathed in the water of God's Holy Word, all the old "tapes" in our minds begin to get cleansed. For our lives to change, we have to soak our lives in truth, loosening up the grime of error and welcoming in what God has called excellent.

Scripture memory sometimes seems impossible. But let the words of Deuteronomy 30:11 ring in our ears: "What I am commanding you today is not too difficult for you or beyond your reach." Scripture memory soars when we create a system that works for our individual personalities. Some people like to write note cards and put them up in places they frequently see, such as in front of a sink. Others listen to Scripture memory tapes. I know many men and women who memorize one verse a week. Over a year they memorize 52 verses. That adds up in a hurry.

Whatever works for you, begin to do it today. We must get the cleansing water of Scripture into our lives.

Feasting by Prayer

Imagine a table set with all your favorite foods. Nothing is bad for you at this table—it's all good for you, and you can satisfy your hunger with the best of fare. This may sound funny in a book about weight loss, but I want to draw a parallel between our relationship with God and the longings we have for fulfillment. Scripture creates this same analogy in Isaiah 55:1-3. "Listen to me, and eat what is good."

Prayer is the table where we feast on the nourishment of our relationship with the Lord. We pray to draw close to the Lord; we also pray that God would show us what's in our hearts. Pray, pray and pray some more.

You see, the solution to changing our lives is not found in behavioral psychology—it's found in the Holy Spirit. We really don't have the power to stop anything. It's the Holy Spirit—gentle and quiet in our lives, with His still, small voice—who creates a new life for us. Let us never think we can ultimately change ourselves; only God can do this, but He needs our permission to do so.

Jeremiah 33:3 says, "Call to me and I will answer you and tell you great and unsearchable things you do not know." God will uncover what is hurt in our lives. First Samuel 16:7 says, "the LORD looks at the heart." Pray to draw close to the Lord, and pray that He would reveal the depths of your heart. When the Lord shows us the issue in our lives, then we can ask for His help in dealing with it. Are our spirits wounded? Ask the Lord to show us where, and pray for healing. Do we need to forgive someone? Ask the Lord to show us who, and then forgive the person. God is faithful. Our invitation is to feast at His table.

Turning the Key of Obedience

We'll cover obedience in greater depth in a later chapter, but I want to touch upon it here. You cannot drive a car unless you first turn it on. You cannot draw close to the Lord except by obedience. John 14:21 says, "Whoever has my commands and obeys them, he is the one who loves me." That doesn't leave much room for discussion. If we know an action that needs to be taken, then we need to take it.

For our emotions to heal, we must follow the pathway of the Lord. His way is right and true, and only when we walk in it, can we experience the life He truly wants us to have.

Is there an area of your life that you know is not obedient to His way? Claim the promise of 1 John 1:9 today—that "if we confess our sins, He is faithful and just and will forgive us our sins and purify us from all unrighteousness."

Resting in His Care

The Lord Jesus wants to use us mightily. He is offering a life better than we could ask for or imagine. But He wants our willingness first. *Stop surviving,* He whispers to us, *and start thriving.* Everyone has experienced trials in life, and trials affect our emotions. But our emotions do not need to rule our lives.

When we stop the destructive self-talk that tells us that we are hopeless and helpless, we can begin to open ourselves to God's way and path. Through Scripture, prayer and obedience, we can walk in the ease of His grace. We can take His yoke upon us, for His burden is easy and His yoke is light.

PART 2:

—SOUL—

We play a big role in how we change, but God plays the ultimate role. He wants our willingness, yet it is only by His power that we grow to be more like Christ.

At the core, the goal of our changing is about bringing glory to the Lord. God desires relationship with us, and as we seek Him, we will find Him—and we will find Him to be greater than anything we could imagine.

This is what we will discuss in the next three chapters.

Stop Wondering; Start Believing

God is good, and He cares for us.
So why do we doubt it?

We do not know what to do, but our eyes are upon you.

2 CHRONICLES 20:12

While driving my usual 45-minute commute from my home on Galveston Bay to the office in Houston, I was listening to Bible teacher Charles Stanley on the radio and taking notes on a napkin. I don't recommend writing while driving a car, but traffic was light, and Pastor Stanley's message was dynamite! (I must confess, I've jotted down some of the most profound thoughts on napkins.)

Pastor Stanley was preaching from 2 Chronicles 20, where the story is told of a vast army of Moabites and Ammonites determined to make war on the people of Judah. Good King Jehoshaphat's resources are vastly outnumbered. Alarmed, the king announces that all the people are to fast—they are to set aside a time of spiritual concentration in order to devote their attention to prayer. As the people come together, Jehoshaphat inquires of the Lord what they should do.

You can feel the tension in the scene. It's horrific. All the men of Judah, with their wives and children, are standing before the Lord. They are silent, expectant, a day or two away from being slaughtered, robbed, raped and enslaved by their enemies. But they pray, waiting for the instruction of their king who has sought the counsel of the King of kings!

As Jehoshaphat cries out to Jehovah, he appeals to the Lord on the basis of God's character. "God," he says, "You rule over all the kingdoms of the nations. Power and might are in your hands" (v. 6). Jehoshaphat reminds the Lord of past faithfulness—"Our God, did you not drive out the inhabitants of this land and give it forever to the descendents of Abraham?" (v. 7). He ends his prayer with one phrase that epitomizes belief in the character and goodness of God. It shows Jehoshaphat's absolute dependence on God, and it shows his absolute faith: "We have no power to face this vast army that is attacking us. We do not know what to do, but our eyes are upon you" (v. 12).

The Lord offers an unexpected solution to Judah's problem and chooses to speak through the prophet Jahaziel. The prophet stands up in that great assembly and encourages the people to believe. "Do not be afraid or discouraged because of this vast army," Jahaziel says. "For the battle is not yours, but God's. . . . You will not have to fight this battle. Take up your positions; stand firm and see the deliverance the LORD will give you" (vv. 15-17).

Do you see God's instruction here? He tells them simply to *stand*.

The next day dawns bright and clear, and as the army of Judah takes the position God has instructed them to take, to their amazement they find that the invading armies have destroyed each other. When Jehoshaphat and all Judah look over the desert toward the vast enemy armies, they see only dead bodies on the ground.

God won the battle. The people only needed to stand and be still.

God, You Know . . .

It's easy to not be still. When trials come our way, we question God's goodness, power, compassion, mercy, tenderness, greatness, gentleness, justice and His ability to make things right.

And trials will come. We are never exempt from pain because we love the Lord. God never promises to spare us from the valley of the shadow of death—He promises to be there in the valley with us and to give us strength for the journey ahead.

How easy it is for us to turn to other solutions before we turn to the Lord. When pain strikes us, our immediate remedy is to turn to whatever offers relief. And what comforts us? The devil presents a striking array of lies to us:

- Food feels so good, so eating more and more of it will surely make you feel better.
- Did God *really* say only one man with one woman? Leave your spouse. He's no good anyway. You'll find love with somebody else for sure.
- You will never succeed, so why even try? Stay at home where it's safe. Never lead. Never risk. Never try.
- When you yell, you are so powerful. No one can hurt you. So you yell at your children, your husband, your boss. There now, doesn't that feel better?

And on and on it goes. Our bad habits are formed when we continually turn to the devil's lies for relief. But those solutions never provide what we so desperately long for. The Bible says that the devil comes to steal, kill and destroy—and we don't have to look hard to see the results of destruction all around us.

Your and my unbelief is always the result of not knowing who God is. When a drunk driver killed our daughter Shari, I had a decision to make. I was devastated. I hurt like I had never hurt before. I had lost my baby who had grown into such a beautiful wife, mother and friend. I could have turned to any number of destructive lies, hoping for relief. But instead, I found myself praying a simple prayer. I'd like to think it was similar to what Jehoshaphat prayed. When Shari was killed, I didn't know what to do. The vast army of her death was more than I could handle. For months I simply prayed, *God, You know* . . .

Those were the only words: *God, You know.* What I meant by this was: *God, You have knowledge. God, You know what's going on. God, You know what to do. And I don't! I have no idea what to do, but my eyes are on You.*

God, You know. It was a simple prayer that encompassed a heart of belief. Our daughter had died, but God was still good. There was no reason I could see for her death, but God knew all there was to it and all there would be. I could see no justice in the situation—it was so random. Why did this happen to our family? But God would make all things beautiful in His time.

God, You know . . .

It is the prayer of belief.

Our unbelief is the groundwork for all that harms us. When we don't believe God, we must place our belief somewhere else. Because all goodness belongs to God, if we have not placed our belief with Him, our belief is placed somewhere that lacks goodness. Our lack of belief causes our destruction. It is because of our unbelief that we tell ourselves that we are horrible parents, dreadful spouses, poor examples to others, bad employees, ineffective leaders.

But we know that a more positive way exists, and we can see something better. There is a solution to our unbelief. It's found in one simple phrase.

What's the phrase?

STOP IT!

Just STOP IT!!!!

STOP IT and STOP IT and STOP IT again.

In this case, stop wondering and start believing. I'm not talking about stopping the good kind of wonder that marvels at something excellent. I'm talking about the destructive type of wonder that causes us to question the character of God. Does God really love me? Does He really care for me? Is God really good? Stop it! Belief is rooted in who God is and what He is like. But we can't believe in someone we don't know. So start getting to know the Lord. Do this by studying the Bible and praying a simple prayer: *Lord, show me who You are.* God is faithful and will reveal His character. I've experienced this.

As We Draw Close

Years ago, I found myself uncertain as to who Jesus was and what He was really like. So for one whole year, I decided to concentrate my Bible reading on only the words of Christ. I used a red-letter edition of the Bible—one that highlights the words of Christ—and pored over everything Christ had to say. I found myself marveling over passages I had read before but had never really internalized.

The shortest verse in the Bible stopped me cold: "Jesus wept" (John 11:35). Why did Christ weep? He was standing at the grave of a close friend, Lazarus, and sorrowing with two dear friends, Mary and Martha. When our own daughter died, the words and the character of Jesus replayed in my mind. "Jesus wept." I could imagine Jesus sorrowing with me—the God of compassion weeping along with me in my loss. Jesus surrounded all of us when Shari died. He knew how much we hurt.

As you and I draw close to the Lord, we can become certain that His way is best. I'm not talking about just head knowledge—I'm talking about the real gut-level knowledge that we act upon. When we believe God, we want what He wants for us. When we believe God, we yield to His good and perfect plan.

Like the people of Judah in the face of an advancing army, we need only to be still.

It's not always easy to be still. I spent 42 years asking God to bless what I was doing. I was living my life—including how I served God—in my own strength. And that is very stressful. In effect, I was saying, I'll change my own character; I'll make myself more like Christ; I'll do great things for God. But I had gotten it backward. That emphasis was all wrong. God alone has the power to do anything. It's not all about me; it's all about God.

In 1984, I yielded control of my life to the Lord. I said, "God, whatever You want for me, wherever I'm supposed to be, whenever You move me—I'm Yours." I had always believed that if I gave Him control, He would send me somewhere I couldn't stand to go or make me do something I couldn't stand to do, but I prayed anyway. It was the prayer of surrender—of belief. I had finally stopped wondering and had started believing that God loves me, wants to use me and ultimately has nothing but goodness in His plans for me.

It hasn't always been easy. The Lord has led my husband, Johnny, and me through some incredible valleys. We've had to declare bankruptcy. We've faced cancer. Our son's home burned to the ground. We've been through the death of a child. Yet God is good—I can say that with every fiber of my being. You know, these days I rarely feel stressed. Yes, I have stressors in my life, but I am seldom worried. God is in control—I know full well that my life is in His hands. Over a period of time, I have come to know the security of belief. I have come to know that God has only good plans for me, and I am more awed by Him every day.

I find great comfort in verses such as Philippians 4:13: "I can do everything through him who gives me strength." The emphasis is on my contentment, not my omnipotence. The power is not mine—it's the Lord's; and my life is secure in the knowledge that I miss out on nothing when I am in His hands.

Another wonderful verse is found in Philippians 3:14: "I press on toward the goal to win the prize for which God has called me heavenward in Christ Jesus." This verse clearly defines my role. My job is to keep pressing on. God's job is to do all the work. In this manner, I can be still. I can believe that He has the power in every circumstance to supernaturally provide for my needs.

When we yield our lives to the Lord, we can truly relax. For years when I prayed, I would offer God various scenarios of how He could answer the prayer. I approached God with a long list of requests, and with the list came suggestions for how He might act! My prayers today mostly concentrate on praising the Lord. I find that when I focus on His character and attributes, the rest of life falls into place. I do pray specific prayers for others and myself—I intercede as Christ interceded when He showed His disciples how to pray. Yet the core of my praying is based on my relationship with the God of the universe. Praying is about spending time with the Lord. He is the One who is all powerful, all knowing, all wise, all loving, all generous, all secure, all safe, all good—and so much more.

When We Stand Firm

What will our lives look like when we, in the same manner as the people of Judah, learn to truly believe and just stand and wait for the Lord? For many of us, the idea of just standing in the face of an oncoming battle sounds like the craziest thing to do. What does it look like when our lives are marked by the firm belief that God is in control?

Have you ever ridden an elevator in a really tall building? That experience is an exercise in belief. When you step inside that little room, you trust that the elevator will do what it says it will do. If you always wondered about the reliability of the elevator and decided to take the stairs instead, that would not be belief. Belief is getting inside the elevator, pushing the button to go to the thirtieth floor, and letting the doors close behind you.

Using this example, we can define belief as an action. When we stand firm, we are not being passive. We are putting our faith into action. Belief is not lying down and letting life wash over us. Belief is stepping in, sitting down, moving forward and pressing on. When we know the Lord, we can rest in Him. Not to confuse you, resting means that we can leap with confidence as we live by faith.

I find that belief provides a certain fearlessness in me. Nothing is too hard to tackle. For instance, I don't like heights. But when I traveled to the Holy Land several years ago, there was no way I was not going to see the top of Masada—the great fortress in the desert where Israel made one last valiant stand against Rome. To get to the top, you can either hike in the hot sun up a windy goat path or take a tramway. I took the tram. (Only one challenge at a time.) I didn't enjoy the height, but I knew that the Lord would not want me to miss this experience. My belief in His goodness and protection enabled me to ride to the top.

Belief also helps me prioritize my involvements and activities. I find that I don't have to say yes to every request that comes my way. I am active in a lot of areas, but I certainly don't believe that God could never get things done without me. I am not indispensable. God is the one who is ultimately responsible for changing lives, not me. When you and I begin to stop wondering and start believing, we may need to give up some activities, even good activities.

Along with believing instead of wondering, I find that rest instead of stress is a huge characteristic of my life. I am content. I wouldn't want to live any other life than mine. So often

I hear in the Christian community about burnout. People get so involved that they wear out for the Lord. Yet I don't see any instruction to do this in Scripture. Jesus offers us an abundant life (see John 10:10), not a worn-out one. No matter what age I am, I know that God will never stop using me for His glory. He has good plans for me as long as I'm around, and I can rest in that knowledge.

Belief also offers us a wealth of joy. This is not the same thing as happiness. Happiness is always based on circumstances. But how can we stay happy when circumstances are always changing? If good things happen, we're happy; if bad things happen, we're not. Joy, however, is the quiet knowledge that all things work together for good when we love God and are called according to His purpose (see Rom. 8:28). When I believe that God loves me, cares about me and has only good planned for me, why would I not want His plan for my life?

The Giver of Good

Belief is at the core of our spiritual life. What we believe about God affects everything. Some people look at God as the great Santa Claus in the sky—someone who doles out toys when we've been nice, and lumps of coal when we've been naughty.

Nothing could be further from the truth. When we discover who God truly is, we find a Being of ultimate glory who opens wide His arms to us. Inside those arms we find grace, love and security. When we come to truly know Him, we can boldly stand firm in the face of any advancing army. We may not know exactly what to do, but we will stand with our faces lifted up and our eyes on Him.

Stop Worrying; Start Trusting

Because we're in God's hands, we have
nothing to worry about—ever!

Faith is being sure of what we hope for.
HEBREWS 11:1

Fact: Some moments in life are just plain bad.

One Christmas holiday season, when our kids were still young, our entire family came down with the flu. Have you ever had everyone in your house sick at the same time? It's horrible. Thermometers get passed back and forth like batons at a track meet. All bathrooms in the house have lineups outside their door. At the best moments, everyone just sort of lies around and groans.

On Christmas Eve we bundled up and went over to my mom's place to celebrate. (What a fun bunch we were.) Christmas day we couldn't even eat a meal, and we stayed sick for days. About a week later, we were so tired of not being able to do anything that we convinced ourselves we were cured. A family celebration was called for. We polled the kids, and for some reason a big bucket of fried chicken won the draw. While Johnny went for take-out, the kids and I excitedly awaited the feast.

Have you ever caught a whiff of fried chicken when you're feeling miserable? Who were we kidding?! That bucket of chicken just sat there in the middle of our table. One by one we excused our-selves and went back to being sick.

Yes, some moments in life are bad, but after enough time has passed, you can laugh—just as I do when I remember all of us morosely sitting around the supper table with a tasty bucket of fried chicken before us, and everyone too sick to even take a bite.

There are plenty of bad moments that aren't nearly as funny. I've had those times, too.

In 1999, my mom grew too frail to care for herself and came to live with Johnny and me. That was hard, but good moments came out of it too. We used to wheel my mom's chair down to the pier so that she could watch the sun setting over the water. She'd watch the sky with its majestic gold and purple hues, and I think she would catch a small glimpse of the glory of heaven that was waiting for her.

Three years later, when we could no longer care for her phys-ically, we needed to place her in a personal care home. Making that kind of decision is one of the most difficult a child will ever make for a parent. Many days I would drive away from the care home crying my eyes out. It felt like I was giving my mom up an inch at a time.

Once, my mom pulled out her feeding tube. The care home called to say an ambulance had taken her to the hospital, and I rushed to be with her. Mom had no idea what had happened. She was fidgety, her hands restless. From 1:00 P.M. until 10:00 P.M. that night, I constantly worked at holding her hands to protect and calm her. It was a surreal moment, caring for my mom who had devoted her life to caring for me. Every time she looked up into my eyes, she'd say, "Oh, Darlin'." My mom couldn't remem-ber my name by then, but she knew I was someone important to her. I feel so privileged to have spent that day with my mom.

When we trust in the Lord, that's the way it is with our bad moments. Romans 8:28 tells us that "in all things God works for the good of those who love him." The Lord has proved this verse to me over and over again. God brings good out of bad—that is the type of God we serve. He knows what He's doing. He loves us, cares for us and makes all things beautiful according to His timetable.

Knowing that, why do we ever worry?

It's a Habit

Sometimes bad experiences really do happen—and sometimes we only *imagine* that bad experiences will happen. In both cases, we worry. When we do, we forget the promises of God. Anxiety comes into our hearts, and our thoughts nag us and cloud the truth. We walk around feeling tense and stressed out. It's hard to see the good in something, particularly when we're smack dab in the midst of a trial.

So why do we worry? Because worry is a convenient response. When our circumstances blind us with pain, worry offers us a handy action. We feel like we're doing something important—we're concerned—and our alarm shows in the furrows on our brow. But worry never solves anything—not one single thing. Worry does nothing except hurt us. It takes our mind off of the Lord and His goodness. It also sends stress hormones throughout the body—telling us to be ready for fight or flight. When we're worried all the time, it's as if our body's motor is revved up but we're not moving anywhere. We're sitting at a stoplight with one foot on the brake and the other foot on the gas pedal.

And still, we worry. The habit is insidious. It sneaks into our lives and fights to control us. It makes us feel numb, in a pit, as if we're drowning. Stop and think about the last time you worried about something. Do you remember what you worried about? Write your thoughts in the following space:

_____

_____

_____

Are you worrying about something right now? If so, there is a solution. A remedy exists to end that destructive pattern in your life so that you can live the life you never dreamed possible—a life filled with meaning and purpose. That life is well within your grasp.

The Stop It Solution

What's the solution?

STOP IT!

Just STOP IT!

STOP IT! and STOP IT and STOP IT again!

You must stop worrying before you can start trusting.

Jesus spoke gentle but strong words about anxiety in Matthew 6. "Do not worry," he said (v. 25). He said that God takes care of the birds of the air and the flowers of the field. Then He asked the rhetorical question, "Are you not much more valuable than they?" (v. 26).

The apostle Paul addressed the subject of worry in Philippians 4:6-7: "Do not be anxious about anything, but in everything, by prayer and petition, with thanksgiving, present your requests to God. And the peace of God, which transcends all understanding, will guard your hearts and your minds in Christ Jesus."

This theme is repeated in 1 Peter 5:7: "Cast all your anxiety on him because he cares for you."

Trust is the confidence that God is good, even when bad things happen. Our lives are in His hands, and we can trust Him, because He has our ultimate good in mind.

This new way of thinking and acting involves two ponents: *our will* and *the Holy Spirit.* First we must decic worrying by consciously and deliberately saying to oursε... ...ιat worry has no place in our lives, and then we must live that way. Then we must depend on *the changing power of the Holy Spirit.* God is ultimately the One who creates lasting good change in our hearts. Yet we play a role in this, too. We have got to want to quit worrying and take steps in that direction. With God as our help, we can do it.

Worry is the direct result of not trusting in the Lord and His goodness. Sure, we all struggle. We all have moments that are literally unbearable—times when we think we can't go through what's in front of us. But worry takes over when we don't believe that the Lord holds all things in His hands or that He loves us, wants the best for us and will one day work all things out for His glory through the circumstances of our lives. When we worry, we are showing unbelief in who God says He is.

Some time ago, a woman came up to me at the end of a First Place conference. She was crying and looked extremely frightened.

"I want to give my life wholeheartedly to the Lord," she said, "but I have five children, all still at home."

"Tell me more of what you mean," I said.

"I'm terribly afraid that God will want to teach me a lesson," she replied. "He'll take one of my children from me, just like He took your daughter Shari from you."

Oh, this poor woman! She had it all wrong! God did not kill my daughter. God doesn't inflict evil on us. Bad things happen because God has set up moral and physical boundaries in this world, and we have to reckon with those boundaries. For instance, God has established the law of gravity. If we get too close to the edge of a cliff and fall off, we have to reckon with the physical reality that our bodies will hit the ground. Regardless of our level of commitment to the Lord, bad things can and do happen to us. But God is able to produce good from bad. Although we get hurt by cruel and senseless things, our God is always kind, compassionate and loving.

Do you trust a God who is always good?

Stop right now to enlist the power of God in your life. Will you pray with me in this area of worry versus trust? Make the prayer personal for your specific experiences.

Lord, You are kind, compassionate and loving. You are always good.
You know that I'm concerned about _____ .
Right now, at this very moment, I want to declare in
prayer that I will not worry about this.
I want to cast all my anxiety upon You, because You care for me.
You are good. You have a plan.
Show me what to do—and what not to do—in this matter.
Help me to trust. I do trust in You.
Amen.

The Bible says that God will prove Himself faithful. Consider the words of Psalm 9:10: "Those who know your name will trust in you, for you, LORD, have never forsaken those who seek you."

A Faith That Trusts

The antidote to worry is to trust the Lord. Another word for trust is "faith." The type of faith I'm talking about is confidence in God. Hebrews 11:1 gives us a definition of that faith: "Faith is being sure of what we hope for and certain of what we do not see." Although we can't tangibly hold our faith in our hands, we know it's there. We can't touch faith or see it with our eyes—yet we know it's real. Trust comes from who we are in Christ. It is our confidence that God is truly who He says He is.

What does this confidence look like? I developed an acronym from the word "faith" to help me remember the remedy to anxiety. Even though the title of this chapter contains the word "trust," think of trust and faith as the same thing in this instance. Trust in the Lord equals **F**earlessly **A**biding **I**n God's **T**ender **H**ands.

F—Fearlessly

Our faith is a *fearless* faith. Second Timothy 1:7 says that "God did not give us a spirit of timidity, but a spirit of power, of love and of self-discipline." Timidity does not come from the Lord, and it has no place in our lives.

Some years ago, I was teaching on 1 Peter 5:8: "Be self-controlled and alert. Your enemy the devil prowls around like a roaring lion looking for someone to devour." Since I don't live in Africa, and I'm not familiar with lions other than those I've seen in the zoo, I did some research.

I found that lions are actually somewhat cowardly. They're not nearly as brave as they appear to be. In fact, the oldest lion in a pride—the frailest, weakest one who has no teeth left—is the lion that has the loudest roar. When a pride stalks prey, they will put the oldest lion on one side of a clearing and all the younger, fiercer lions on the other side. As the prey comes through the clearing, the oldest lion will roar his loudest, scaring the prey toward the others. What a picture of our fear!

The next verse (1 Pet. 5:9) goes on to say, "Resist [the enemy], standing firm in the faith." When we trust the Lord, we have nothing to be afraid of.

A—Abiding

"Abiding" is a somewhat old-fashioned word. It means to continue or to stay close. Its antonyms are "avoid, depart, move, reject, resist." I love how the *King James Version* puts John 15:4-5—we are to abide in Christ. We cannot flourish except when we are closely connected to Him.

Have you ever been in the opposite place of abiding? When you are not abiding in Christ, you avoid Him. You try to quench your hunger or thirst with something that is destructive to your life.

But when you abide in Christ, you stay close to Him, no matter what you are going through. Even when you are going through painful times, that's when clinging to Christ is of utmost importance. It may hurt like crazy, but often it's in the painful places that we learn the most valuable lessons.

I—In God's

We must place our trust nowhere else but in God. People profess faith in all sorts of things that will ultimately fail them—money, spirituality, technology, science, themselves.

I read an article in the *Houston Chronicle* recently about an author who had written a book on faith. There was not one mention of God. To me, that kind of book is worthless. You can't separate true faith from the Lord. Only when we know who God is can we trust Him. Only when we are confident of the character of the Lord can we have real peace.

John 14:6 records that Christ is "the way and the truth and the life." Our faith must be placed in Him and Him alone.

T—Tender

The Lord Jesus is gentle and patient with us. Isaiah 40:11 describes the Lord as someone who "tends his flock like a shepherd: He gathers the lambs in his arms and carries them close to his heart; he gently leads those that have young." What a beautiful picture of how the Lord acts toward us! When we trust the tenderness of the Lord, we can have confidence that He will act with compassion toward us.

A woman named Miriam came to one of our Bible classes at church. Miriam was anorexic and weighed about 90 pounds. She hated God and wanted nothing to do with Him, but she was led to the church by a sense that she needed to talk with Beth Moore, a national Bible teacher who is also a member of our church.

Miriam wasn't able to talk to Beth, who was away, but she stayed for a class. Afterward, two of the sweetest senior-aged women in the church invited her for lunch. Miriam told me later that she simply couldn't say no. As the women prepared the meal, Miriam felt a sense of tenderness she had not felt in a long, long time. Even though Miriam was anorexic, the gentleness of the women drew her in and she ate lunch with them because they had prepared it with their own hands especially for her.

God is tender when we suffer. The Lord knew exactly what Miriam needed to be drawn to the truth of His love for her.

H—Hands

I love the words of Isaiah 49:16. The Lord says, "See, I have engraved you on the palms of my hands." Can you imagine that? God cares for us so much that He has tattooed our names where He can constantly see them. We are in God's hands. He sees every need we are facing today. He will strengthen and help us. "I will uphold you with my righteous right hand," He says in Isaiah 41:10. That's what our trust is all about. God has us in His hands. We have nothing to worry about—ever.

A Powerful and Effective Remedy

What is the antidote to worry? Trust. It means that we have a confidence that fearlessly abides in God's tender hands. The Bible says that we "do not have, because [we] do not ask" (Jas. 4:2). If you really want to have trust, you only need to ask Him.

When you trust the Lord, you are able to believe God for bigger things than you could ever imagine. That trust will look different for different people. It may simply mean having enough strength to go for a walk or to get up and clean your house. God is tender with us. He knows exactly where each of us are and where we need to be.

If you are worrying about something right now, in its place you can find trust if you are willing to place your confidence in the goodness of the Lord.

CHAPTER 7

Stop Wavering; Start Obeying

If we say that we love God, we need to obey Him.

Now what I am commanding you today is not too difficult for you or beyond your reach.

DEUTERONOMY 30:11

In 1979, my mom and I took the trip of a lifetime. Little did I know this trip was something the Lord would use to teach me about obedience.

My mom and I were part of a church choir that toured parts of Europe. We traveled through England, Scotland, Ireland and Wales. We performed 14 concerts in 14 days. It was a whirlwind of activity. We saw huge gray cathedrals and wonderful old cobblestone streets. We met believers from around the world who loved the same Lord we did. We sang our hearts out at each concert.

Our nearly perfect trip was marred by only one thing. Toward the end, one of the leaders informed us the trip had gone over budget and each person would need to pay an extra $200. Nobody was happy about that. My mom had paid for both of our trips, so that meant an extra $400 for her. That was a lot of money for anyone in 1979. I offered to pay. But somehow, that check never got written. I couldn't tell you why. I guess it slipped my mind. When you're on a trip, there's a lot to think about. But the truth is, I'm not a detail person, and I should have made a note of it. I should have done what I promised.

Twenty years went by. One day, I suddenly remembered what I said I would do. Oh, how I rationalized! *Good grief,* I thought, *it has been two decades. The trip's long since been paid for. They should have calculated the right price in the first place. I'm not even sure how to reach the travel hosts. Maybe they're not even around anymore. This is just embarrassing. There's late and then there's LATE.*

I stewed and I fumed, but I knew the Holy Spirit was working on me. The Living God was telling me I needed to do something—and I was wavering. It didn't matter how silly or trivial it may have seemed to me. I owed somebody money. I needed to make my account right with God by making my account right with man. The question was whether or not I would obey.

Has that ever happened to you? Have you ever found yourself in a place where you know you need to do something, but you don't want to do it? Maybe doing it makes you feel a bit awkward, or it's a difficult or scary thing—so you think up all sorts of reasons to get out of doing it. Life will continue—sometimes for days, weeks or even years—with periodic reminders flashing through your mind of what you know you need to do. The thought simply will not leave you alone. No matter how you try to shake yourself free, the pressure to do what's right is always there. The Holy Spirit sure can be relentless.

I wrote that check 20 years later—for $500. (There had to be some kind of interest, right?) I tracked down the tour hosts and mailed them the money, along with a letter of apology. They wrote back and thanked me. They had forgotten about it and probably never would have remembered.

But that didn't matter. The test was mine to pass.

It's Easy to Waver

Hebrews 12:1 describes sin as something that "so easily entangles" us. When we're faced with a difficult decision or action, it's easy to waver.

Most of us don't get excited about the thought of obedience. One of the definitions of the word "obey" is to comply, to behave, to follow commands or guidance. That's not the easiest thing to do. Have you ever watched a mother telling her three-year-old daughter to keep her voice down indoors, to not run out in the street, to not draw on the walls—or any of the hundreds of other instructions parents have to give their children? Obedience is not something we naturally do when we're children, and it's not always the path we follow when we're grown up either.

I think there's something in us that innately resists being told what to do, even though we know it's good for us. The apostle Paul expressed this struggle so perfectly in Romans 7:15. He admitted that he had no idea why he kept messing up—he just did. "I do not understand what I do," he wrote. "For what I want to do I do not do, but what I hate I do." Can you relate to that? Is there some behavior in your life that you hate but still keep doing? A bad habit is like that.

Think about your life for a moment. Do any of the following apply?

- Overeating is not good for you. Yet a dozen donuts are right in front of you, so you eat the whole box.
- Moving around is good for you, yet you settle in on the couch instead of going for a walk.
- Spending time each day with the Lord through prayer and Scripture reading is required if you want to know the Lord better and learn to trust and obey Him. Yet when the alarm goes off, you hit the snooze button— again and again and again.

Joshua 24:14-15 records a classic struggle between wavering and obedience. "Now fear the LORD and serve him with all faithfulness," Joshua instructs the Israelites. "But if serving the LORD seems undesirable to you, then choose for yourselves this day whom you will serve."

It's easy to waver when it comes to sin. Truth lies before us—we know what to do, or what not to do—and yet we hesitate. Can you hear the words of Joshua in your ear today? "Choose for yourself whom you will serve."

God knows that obedience is difficult. Still, He instructs His people to walk in paths that are good and not harmful. He knows that obedience to His loving instructions brings us hope, purpose, peace and health. Equally so, God knows that if certain of His promises are disobeyed, the results are never beneficial to us.

What happens when we do not obey the Lord? We reap the natural consequences of our harmful behavior.

- Despair, fear and anxiety are much more prevalent in our lives.
- We never get what we hope for—sin always lies; it never satisfies.
- We lose respect for ourselves.
- We find it difficult to set an example for our children, our grandchildren and others who look to us for guidance.
- We lose interest in attending church and being around other believers, in reading God's Word or in praying.
- Our consciences know the truth of our disobedience, and that knowledge weighs on us, making our lives miserable.
- Our prayers are not as effective.
- Our relationships are not as free of conflict.

God always loves us, even when we sin. When we do sin, even though God's arms are open wide to receive us, He wants us to obey Him so that He can open up the full extent of His blessings for us. When we truly obey Him—when we follow His pathways wholeheartedly—we are able to have the full relationship with Him that we so desperately long for. We are able to have the amazing lives that He fully intends for us to have.

Think of wavering versus obeying like this: You're out on a summer hike, carrying a big canteen of water. If you drink it, it will completely do what it is intended to do—quench your thirst.

What happens if some dirt gets mixed into the water? A few specks begin to make the water cloudy. The water is still useful, but not as effective as it could be. When more dirt is added, the canteen becomes heavier, the water more unpleasant. It's still water; it's just not the sparkling, pure water it could be.

Sin in our lives is like dirt mixed into a canteen of water. When we sin, we are still loved by the Lord—that is a fact that never changes—but our lives become murky and impure.

A Life of Promise

There is a better way. Change is within our reach. It is possible to stop wavering when it comes to sin and start obeying the Lord. But God needs our cooperation.

What's the solution?

We've got to STOP IT!!

We've got to stop wavering between good and evil and choose the pathway toward which the Lord is directing us. We must take responsibility to stop the bad on the way to starting the good.

Our life's calling is to be healthy, whole people who live victoriously and with a sense of purpose. The Lord knows that without a healthy life, we're going to be miserable inside and out. In order to live with health, we must be committed to the process of change the same way an athlete commits to preparing for a race. We must want to change and ask the Lord to help us change. When we step out in obedience, we will be amazed at the life that opens up to us.

Living obediently is not without its challenges. Destructive habits can become ingrained in us to such an extent that they feel normal after a while. When we stop the bad habits and replace them with positive ones, it may take some time before we have fully adjusted to the new good habit of obedience. But we can start today.

There are at least two reasons why obeying the Lord is of utmost importance: first, it's the way we tell Him we love Him. Second, it's the catalyst for receiving His love and care for us.

Obedience Is God's Love Language

The predominant way we can tell the Lord that we love Him is not by doing things for Him, giving things to Him, praising Him or spending time with Him. Those are all beneficial, but none of those communicate the way Christ asks to be loved.

Jesus said, If you love me, you will do what I command (see John 15:14). He isn't being egotistical. He's the Son of God, the second member of the Trinity—the very nature and substance of the everlasting Lord of the universe. Love and obedience go hand in hand. Jesus is saying that there is a condition to calling ourselves Christians—if we say that we love Him, then we must obey Him. We must honor the pathways He has set for us. There is no other way.

Obedience is God's love language. When we're obedient to Him, we're telling God that He's our boss, our commander-in-chief, our Lord. We're saying that we believe He is who He says He is.

Obedience Is Good for Us

Obedience becomes much easier for us when we start to believe that God only has good in mind for us. He wants to bless us, to restore our health, our families, our finances and our relationships. (Sometimes our good means experiencing correction, but the pain of correction always results in what is best for us.)

We tend to think of God's commandments as a long list of harsh rules to follow. Somehow, if we step out of line, God will give us a swat with His supernatural kitchen spoon. But when we start to examine the commandments of God as found in Scripture, we find that they are always given with our best interests in mind. God's commandments are never arbitrary. They always have a purpose. And that purpose nurtures and cares for us.

Perhaps it's easier to think of God's commands as promises to us. Even though "promise" is a gentler word than "command," there is still obedience involved. Just check out some of His promises and the benefits for us if we obey.

- If we confess our sins, He will forgive them (see 1 John 1:9).
- If we come to Him when we are weary, He will give us rest (see Matt. 11:28).
- If we wait on the Lord, He will renew our strength (see Isa. 40:31).
- If we delight ourselves in Him, He will give us the desires of our hearts (see Ps. 37:4).
- If we forgive others, God will forgive us (see Matt. 6:14).
- If we cast our anxiety on Him, He will give us peace (see Phil. 4:6-7).

It is imperative for us to obey the Lord—not only to show Him love but also because it is good for us. As we obey God, He is able to bring about His good plan for our lives.

Saying "Yes, Lord"

What area of obedience is the Lord calling you to address today?

Perhaps He wants you to say yes to an opportunity you've been saying no to, or He wants you to fully yield your life to Him.

Perhaps He wants you to talk to someone you don't want to talk to, or stop a destructive habit that is harming you, or change an attitude, or start a health plan, or throw something out, or rest in Him instead of worrying.

Obedience can take a lot of different forms.

My parents became Christians and were baptized when I was six years old. I also wanted to be baptized. When our pastor talked with me, I must have given him the answers he wanted to hear, but truly I had no idea what I was doing. I remember coming up out of the water saying, "That was fun," but I didn't really understand.

I believe the Bible teaches that baptism is an outward symbol of our new life in Christ. When we get baptized—when we go under the water and come up out of it—we are symbolically buried with Him and resurrected to a new life. Baptism doesn't save us, but it's something that Christ instructs us to do as a way of telling others we've put our trust in Him.

When I was 12 years old, I accepted Jesus into my heart and became a Christian. I knew in my heart that I should be baptized again, since I hadn't truly understood what baptism meant when I was 6 years old. However, I was told that I should just rededicate my life, so I didn't follow through with baptism.

The thought of getting baptized—with full knowledge this time—never went away completely. I knew that my desire was the Holy Spirit wanting me to be obedient. Years went by. Johnny and I got married and started our family. We became active in our church. Finally, when I was 29, I stopped wavering about this area of obedience. I must confess that the thought of getting baptized didn't thrill me. Our three children were 11, 9 and 7 by then. I taught a sixth-grade Sunday School class. I was the one who was supposed to have my spiritual ducks in a row. I had to be obedient.

And do you know what? It wasn't that bad after all.

The time to stop wavering is now. God's will for each of us is that we obey Him. Obedience begins when we say yes to the Lord.

God's plans for us are always good, and they include hope and a bright future.

PART 3:

—MIND—

Our minds are where we think, perceive, plan and reason. Our minds can affect so much of our lives—everything from what type of mood we're in, to what sort of decisions we make.

The battle for our minds has never been greater than it is today. Our minds are constantly bombarded with thoughts of how to think and live. We must depend on God's Holy Word to guide our minds in paths of righteousness. By His power we will grow to be more like Christ every day.

That's what the next three chapters will discuss.

Stop Indulging;
Start Considering

We can give in to every urge, or we can
focus on the consequences.
One way leads to hurt, the other way to health.

*In the spring, at the time when kings go off to war, David sent Joab out
with the king's men and the whole Israelite army.*

2 SAMUEL 11:1

The storyteller begins this account on an ominous note, almost as
if preparing us for the tragedy about to unfold: "In the spring, at
the time when kings go off to war, David sent Joab out" (2 Sam.
11:1).

Did you catch what it says?

David sent Joab out *in his place.*

After the harshness of winter was over, it was customary for
kings in the historic Middle East to resume military maneuvers.
Regardless of our beliefs about war today, this was what kings
were supposed to do back then—protect and defend their people
and their country's interests. As king of Israel, that was David's
God-given assignment. Yet David sent Joab instead. And that
was David's first mistake. He assigned someone else to do what
God had clearly called him to do. David's will replaced God's

plan and purpose for David's life. Self-will is always at the root of self-indulgence. When we choose the first, we automatically choose the second.

After years of hiding from Saul—on the run in the desert and living in caves—David had finally taken his rightful place as king of Israel. He was living in the palace, a very comfortable place to reside. But in his comfort and leisure, David forgot that along with privilege comes responsibility. Now living in luxury, David had forgotten the God who sustained him, protected him and anointed him king. He began to use his position and power to establish a pattern that would lead to destruction. He wasn't thinking of the long-term; he was living without considering the consequences. As the story unfolds, we see the results of David's initial folly. While Joab was out fighting wars, David was enjoying the pleasures of the flesh.

When we look at what David would later use—food and drink—to try to trick Uriah the Hittite into going home to his wife to cover the fact that David had slept with her and she had conceived, it is highly possible that part of David's self-indulgence that fateful evening when he saw Bathsheba bathing was a lavish meal and lots of wine. After his meal, David decided to take a stroll on the palace rooftop, perhaps needing some fresh air after an overindulgent meal. While he was on the rooftop, David saw a woman taking a bath. He indulged his eyes by feasting on her beauty. Do you begin to see a pattern here? First David indulges himself in the luxuries of the palace rather than going to war. Then he probably indulges in a banquet-type meal; then he indulges his eyes on forbidden pleasures. Before long we will see him indulge in other pleasures clearly forbidden in God's law.

If David, the man after God's own heart, could succumb to such self-indulgent behavior, we are foolish to think we can indulge one of our senses and refrain from temptation to indulge in other ways!

It is easy to read about David's encounter with Bathsheba and think that she was a stranger when David summoned her for an evening of temporary pleasure. However, by reading the genealogies (those parts of the Bible we tend to skip over), we learn that Bathsheba was the granddaughter of Ahithophel, one of David's most trusted advisors. To even consider defiling this young woman was an affront to David's dear friend! And to make matters even worse, Bathsheba was a married woman—the wife of one of David's loyal commanders. If in his drunken state David did not remember who this young woman was, a servant tactfully asked him, "Isn't this Bathsheba, the daughter of Eliam and the wife of Uriah the Hittite?" (v. 3). Driven by a self-indulgent mentality, David ignored that still, small voice that invited him to STOP IT! before it was too late. (Before you pass judgment on David, ask yourself how many times you have ignored God's still, small voice as you raced swiftly toward certain destruction.)

The situation went from bad to worse. After a one-night stand, Bathsheba discovered that she was pregnant. So David scrambled to cover his indiscretion. He asked Bathsheba's husband, Uriah, to come home from war, hoping that Uriah would sleep with his wife while he was home—then the child would look like it was Uriah's, not David's.

But Uriah proves too noble for that. He was not tricked into abandoning his responsibility to the men he commanded by indulging himself with fine food and abundant wine and an evening of pleasure with his wife. "The ark and Israel and Judah are staying in tents," Uriah told David, "and my master Joab and my lord's men are camped in the open fields. How could I go to my house to eat and drink and lie with my wife? As surely as you live, I will not do such a thing!" (v. 11).

Unable to persuade Uriah to go home, David decided to indulge another sense—his sense of pride. Rather than admitting what he had done, David plotted to have Uriah killed so that he could marry Bathsheba and pretend that everything was right in his self-indulgent little world. However, there is one problem David didn't bargain for. It is spelled out in 2 Samuel 11:27: "The thing David had done displeased the LORD." What a chilling verse!

One bad choice led to another—David chose to shirk his responsibility, and now he had committed murder.

Through the prophet Nathan, the Lord rebuked King David. Nathan prophesied the end result of David's sin—the child that David and Bathsheba had conceived would become sick and die. Nathan also predicted "the sword will never depart from [David's] house" (2 Sam. 12:10). True to Nathan's prophecy, David and Bathsheba's child became sick and died. As history shows, Nathan's prophecy about David's house never having peace came to pass as well.

In one evening of living to indulge his senses—the day he decided to stay home in the spring instead of doing what he was supposed to do—one indulgence led to another like a snowball gaining speed downhill until David had fallen into a grievous sin pattern that would haunt him for the rest of his life. Because David did not STOP IT! before it began, the thing he had done displeased the Lord.

What a tragic story, and what a lesson for us!

The Problem with Temporary Pleasure

It's a funny thing when we start making wrong choices: There's no end to the chaos that living to indulge can create.

Imagine you're at home watching television for an evening. How many commercials would you typically see in the course of three hours? Can you imagine if you did everything that every commercial told you to do for just one day?

You'd need to buy four or five new cars—maybe more.

You'd need to eat at a string of fast-food restaurants.

You'd have to fill the trunk of one of your new cars with cases of cola, new carpeting for your house, two or three mattresses, the paperwork for several credit card offers, a half-dozen pairs of athletic shoes, one set of amazing Ginsu knives and one Culligan man.

And that's just in one night!

We live in a world that caters to our inclination to indulge ourselves. That's why all those candy bars and tabloid magazines are placed at the checkout counter of the grocery store. The pressure is ever present to give in to our cravings. If there's an itch, we and others will convince ourselves that we need to scratch it.

Most of our destructive habits do not spring from our logic—we don't do these things because we've thought them out fully and made a plan of action based on considering the consequences. Destructive habits arise because we choose behaviors based on our whims. We act out of a presumed need to gratify ourselves—a need to satisfy a longing right now and usually without thinking. That's why advertisers bombard us with their messages.

My friend Elizabeth Crews works as an addictions counselor. She tells me that most people get caught in their destructive patterns of behavior because they focus only on the temporary pleasure of the moment. If life turns sour in any way, people too often seek the temporary good feelings brought about by their harmful behavior. It's the thrill of a joy ride. It's the dubious pleasure of a 20-minute rush.

What is your indulgence? What is the craving that calls to you again and again? What is the pattern that causes hurt and harm in your life?

Perhaps it's overeating. You don't think about it—you just do it. When the going gets tough—and that seems to happen most days—you reach for the bag of popcorn or the package of cookies and keep going.

Maybe it's anger. You can flare up anytime—while driving, while talking on the phone to your kids or coworkers. It seems like the slightest spark will ignite a fire within you.

Perhaps your indulgence is shopping. Whenever you're at a store, it seems as though you just can't say no to purchasing something. There's always a "good" excuse—the store is having a sale, you need to stock up on something, or you just need a pick-me-up. At the end of the month, however, your outgo is more than your income.

These are the momentary pleasures that lead to our destruction. These are the patterns that make us miserable. These behaviors never result in what we hope they will bring—they never result in lasting peace, joy, purpose, satisfaction, hope or health.

These behaviors are traps set by the enemy. They are snares that steal from us, kill our spirits and destroy our lives.

But there is a solution.

Play the Tape

What's the remedy?

STOP IT!

Just STOP IT!

STOP IT and STOP IT and STOP IT again.

In this case, we must stop our indulging and start our considering. We have to look past the temporary pleasure of the moment and take time to consider where a particular behavior will lead. Instead of focusing on the high we get from our destructive behavior—whether overeating, substance abuse, pornography, shopping, gambling, being overly busy, or whatever it is—we need to stop long enough to see the predictable consequences of our behavior.

Let's take stock right now of a few possible consequences. We won't focus on the momentary indulgence but on the long-term results of the indulgence.

- Overeating leads to a host of poor health problems—high blood pressure, diabetes, heart disease—and social problems—not fitting in an airplane seat without a seat-belt extender, not wanting to put on a swimsuit, not being able to join others in activities that require some physical exertion—and lower self-esteem and lack of self-respect.
- Overspending leads to debt, arguments and blame between spouses, less money for necessities, and sometimes even bankruptcy.
- Drinking too much can lead to embarrassment, liver disease, DUIs, fines, loss of a driver's license, injury, death, prison time.

Are any of these consequences reflected in your life? Can you name some personal consequences not listed? Sometimes we're hesitant to call a problem a problem or to admit that we have a problem in the first place. But a problem is a problem if it interferes with our lives. Is something hindering your marriage? Your relationship with your kids? Your productivity at work? Your relationships at church? Then that's a problem.

Your situation is not hopeless. Stopping your destructive thoughts and actions has the power to open up a life you never dreamed possible—a life filled with meaning and purpose. This good life is well within your grasp. But you must first stop the bad on the way to starting the good.

One of the tools that Elizabeth Crews gives to recovering alcoholics and drug addicts is the admonition to "play the tape all the way through." Instead of indulging, Elizabeth asks them to look past the temporary pleasure of the moment and take the time to consider where that particular behavior will lead. They are asked to look past the transitory good feelings and to focus on the not-so-pleasant end results.

For instance, instead of seeking the thrill of drinking too much, they are asked to stop and imagine the shame, remorse and guilt of letting themselves and their loved ones down—one more time. They are urged to consider the damage they may cause to their car, to people's lives, or the months they may spend behind prison bars.

Then they are asked to play another tape all the way through. Elizabeth suggests that they picture themselves resisting the temptation to fall back into the old behavior. They are asked to visualize how good they will feel when they graduate from an in-patient program, when they receive a 10-year sobriety token, when they can hold their head high and give good advice to others struggling with addiction.

Playing the tape through is a powerful tool when combating the immediate-gratification disease known as addiction.

I believe that playing the tape all the way through is excellent advice for anybody struggling with patterns of destructive behavior. When temptation comes, one of the God-given ways of escaping the snare is to stop long enough to picture the end results.

For example, when it comes to overeating, instead of focusing on how good the food will taste, we can picture the predictable results. We can see ourselves weighing in during our weight-loss meeting and having to make excuses for our lack of progress. We can feel the disappointment we will experience because, once again, we have let ourselves down. We can picture having to write this failing in our prayer journal.

Or, we can play another tape.

In this case, we can picture how we will feel if we resist the temptation to overeat. We feel the joy of sharing our victory at our next weight-loss meeting. We visualize holding our head high as we tell our story to others just beginning their journey toward health.

Playing the tape through is a valuable weapon that allows us to use our imaginations in a way that brings glory to God and success to our lives. What tapes can you play in your life? Take a moment to play a couple right now. You may want to jot some thoughts in the space below:

*I consistently struggle with the following bad habit:*_____
_____.

*When I play the tape through, the end result of this habit makes me feel*_____;

does the following to my self-respect: _____
_____;

typically produces the following results in me: _____
_____ *and*
can affect other people by _____.

*If left unchecked, this behavior will probably lead to the following long-term consequences :*_____
_____

If I play the other tape all the way through and choose not to give in to my bad habit,
I feel _____;

my self-respect is _____;

*typically produces the following results in me:*_____
_____;

and can affect other people by _____ .

If I keep away from this bad habit, I will benefit from the following long-term results: _____

_____ .

In Deuteronomy 30:19-20, Moses summoned all the Israelites together and asked them to renew their commitment to the Lord: "This day I call heaven and earth as witnesses against you that I have set before you life and death, blessings and curses. Now choose life, so that you and your children may live and that you may love the LORD your God, listen to his voice, and hold fast to him."

That choice is ours today. Life and death are before us. Let us choose life in such a way that we and our loved ones may live. Let us love God, listen to His voice and hold fast to Him.

Let us stop indulging and start considering.

God Can Change Your Trajectory

"Trajectory" is a word we don't often use. But I want us to remember it here. It may sound silly, but I encourage you to say it out loud several times in order to plant it in your mind.

Trajectory.

Picture the curve an object makes as it leaves one location and heads toward another. That's a trajectory. A trajectory is a route, course or flight path. A tennis ball creates a trajectory when it is lobbed over the net. A missile follows a trajectory when it is launched from a ship toward an enemy target. Applying the concept of trajectory to the events of our lives, when events get set in motion at one place, they happen in another.

Our lives have trajectory. The decisions we make today will affect our future. Every choice we make yields a result. When we choose to engage in harmful behaviors, we set in motion events that will produce outcomes somewhere else. What trajectory are you on right now?

Giving in to your impulses creates one set of results. Focusing on the consequences enables you to make better choices that lead to positive results. Your task is to stop indulging and start considering—thinking of where every choice will lead.

One wonderful thing about our Lord is that He is able to change the trajectory we are on. No matter what decisions we have made in the past, we are not doomed to destruction in the future. God promises that He will complete the good work He began in us when we committed our lives to Him. Isaiah 1:18 offers a wonderful promise: "Though your sins are like scarlet," says the Lord, "they will be white as snow; though they are red as crimson, they shall be like wool."

I mentioned this earlier, in chapter 6: Changing your life involves two key components. The first is your will. You have to firmly decide to take a plan of action, however small or large it may be, and then do it. Second, you have to depend on the changing power of the Holy Spirit in your life. God is ultimately the One who creates lasting, good change in your heart and life. God changes you, yet you also play a role in this, and neither role can be ignored. You've got to want to change and then take steps in that direction.

I find 1 Timothy 6:11-12 to be a tremendous instruction in this area: "But you, man [woman] of God, flee from all this, and pursue righteousness, godliness, faith, love, endurance and gentleness. Fight the good fight of the faith. Take hold of the eternal life to which you were called."

Our trajectories are not set in stone.

With God's power and our willingness, a new life can be ours.

Stop Absorbing; Start Discerning

Embracing everything that comes our way is
a sure track to a cluttered mind.
Filtering life through God's Word produces
a clear view of reality.

Does not wisdom call out? Does not understanding raise her voice?

PROVERBS 8:1

Have you ever heard the saying that we are to be *in* the world but not *of* the world?

What does that mean?

It means that we need to live here on planet Earth, along with all the customs and ways of life that make us human. We're not called to live life in a vacuum with huge barriers that isolate us from the people around us. We're to be *in* the world. God has us here for a specific reason: to interact with people who need to know about God's grace and love, and to enjoy the Lord forever.

But we're not *of* the world either. This world is not our true home. We move around in it, yes, but we're not bound to it—we don't give the world the same allegiance that we give to the Lord.

Let's put this in everyday terms.

What would happen if I showed up one Monday morning at work wearing just any old thing I felt like wearing? Can you picture it? I'd open the door to the offices at First Place, wave a cheery hello to my colleague Nancy Taylor and waltz to my desk, perhaps wearing patched blue jeans with paint splotches and one of Johnny's old work shirts and with my hair not done. Or maybe I'd feel like coming into the office dressed like my granddaughters when they were five—in whatever suited their fancy at the moment. I could wear a ballerina tutu, my pajamas, or a bathing suit. How well do you think that would go over?

Here's the truth: Because I'm called to be *in* the world, my culture dictates that I show up at work wearing clothes suitable for a professional office environment. Women's fashion is so broad these days; there's a lot of leeway in what "professional" looks like. But regardless of the choices, there is a cultural expectation that those who work in an office should look polished and coordinated when they arrive at their desk on Monday morning. We need to live within our culture. And that's okay.

Suppose I worked in an office where the culture encouraged all of its employees to cheat on their taxes, take three-hour lunch breaks while still on the clock, and flirt with their married bosses. What would I do then?

In that case, I must say no to my culture. I'm *in* it, but not *of* it. That means I don't have to participate in unethical or immoral activities. I'm called to discern truth from error and live in such a way that pleases the King of kings and Lord of lords. I must discern how to live on this earth.

Culture itself is not the enemy, but some of the ideas and behaviors within a culture cannot be taken lightly. If we absorb everything that comes our way without discernment, we're in danger of absorbing a whole lot of harmful stuff.

What happens if we don't filter our culture through the Word of God? What happens if we accept every message that comes our way?

A Cluttered Mind

Can you picture a trashcan that needs to be emptied?

That's our mind when we don't filter our culture through a biblical worldview.

Our culture is all around us. Whenever we talk with a neighbor, we're interacting with culture. Whenever we read a magazine, listen to a song, go to a movie, watch TV or read a book, we're interacting with culture. Whenever we go to work or school or the shopping center, we're interacting with culture. In this sense, culture is neither bad nor good; it's neither enemy nor friend. Culture is a morally neutral medium, like water, food or trees.

But because the concept of culture is morally neutral, culture can be used for bad or for good purposes. Right now you're reading a book—a method of communicating that is part of our culture. A book can be used for a variety of purposes: to promote health and vitality or to incite a population to violence. Culture can steal, kill and destroy us, or it can be used to bring health, healing and wholeness.

Below are some messages heard in our culture today. These messages could come to you via television, a magazine or newspaper, a friend, a conference speaker, a coworker, your mother—it doesn't really matter where the information comes from. Are the following messages harmful or beneficial, or could they be harmful or beneficial depending to what degree a person follows them?

- To be a good parent, you must give your child everything she wants.
- Every time you feel pain, you should take pills.
- Women absolutely can't look their age. Looking older is the same thing as looking unattractive.

- After a hard day's work, your reward should be a bowl of ice cream.
- If your marriage isn't working, you should look for a better partner.
- The way to start your family's day is with fun, and that means stopping for donuts on the way to school.

As you considered each statement and filtered the truth from error, you were exercising the skill of discernment. Proverbs 2:11 states that "discretion will protect you, and understanding will guard you." We are called to be wise—to have our minds in tune with truth. We can't pretend that evil doesn't exist; we need to recognize evil for what it is. We're also called to embrace understanding and sound judgment. We are to know the truth, for the truth sets us free (see John 8:32).

When we accept every message brought forth from our culture, we are susceptible to every whim any huckster can dream up. We become unstable, tossed back and forth by whatever we see and hear. We absorb ideas that can hurt our bodies and make our souls sad, our spirits sick and our thoughts a confused mess.

There are some good messages in our culture today, but there are also a pack of lies. When we believe lies, our lives follow suit. We end up in destructive patterns that seem to have no end. Those destructive areas of our lives affect who we are, what we tell ourselves, what we think and how we act. We end up whispering to ourselves things such as:

- I'm a horrible mother (father).
- I'm a dreadful wife (husband).
- I'm not a good example to others.
- I'm a bad employee.
- I'm an awful leader.

Stop for a moment and take a breath after all you have just read. Know that your situation is not hopeless. A more positive way exists. You know this. You can see something better. Deep down, you long to be the kind of person you admire. You can picture him or her right now. You're picturing a person who has more patience than you do, more joy, peace or happiness. This is a person who doesn't quit, who doesn't lose her temper, who never gives up, whose life is characterized by discipline and satisfaction.

There is a way to become that person. That's right; you know what I'm going to say. What's the solution?

STOP IT!

Just STOP IT!!!

STOP IT and STOP IT and STOP IT again!!!

In this case, *stop absorbing* and *start discerning*.

Stop absorbing means that we stop believing every message we hear from our culture. We stop taking in as truth everything we see, hear or read. Just because some expert wrote something in a magazine doesn't mean that we have to live our lives according to the pattern of what he or she declared as truth. Just because some celebrity acted a certain way in a movie doesn't mean we need to do the same thing if the same situation arises in our life. Just because a friend swears by a certain remedy doesn't mean it will be good for us. We need to stop convincing ourselves that our children must have everything they tell us they must have. We must stop responding to all the lies that come our way in the mail. We must stop surfing all the garbage on the Internet that's put on display and is so easily accessible.

Just STOP IT!!

The Bible Solution

First Corinthians 13:11 records these words: "When I was a child, I talked like a child, I thought like a child, I reasoned like a child. When I became a man [or woman], I put childish ways behind me." The time to start thinking like a grownup is now. As grownups, we must start filtering our culture through the Word of God. When the Word of God gets into our lives it acts as a cleansing and purifying agent. The Word of God leads and guides us. The Word of God acts as a safeguard. When we immerse ourselves in the Bible, we immerse ourselves in the very thoughts of a holy and righteous God.

Consider the cry of David in Psalm 119:68. He points to the character of God and the need to have the thoughts of God in his life. "You are good," David says to God, "and what you do is good; teach me your decrees."

The words of Joshua 1:8 exhort us to dig deeply into Scripture: "Do not let this Book of the Law depart from your mouth; meditate on it day and night, so that you may be careful to do everything written in it. Then you will be prosperous and successful."

Second Timothy 3:16-17 gives us the promise that "all Scripture is God-breathed and useful for teaching, rebuking, correcting and training in righteousness, so that the man of God may be thoroughly equipped for every good work."

Ultimately, we read Scripture to get closer to the Lord. As we dig deeply into the Word of God, we come to know the very character of the One who is infinitely wise, infinitely discerning, infinitely beneficial and infinitely good. "Taste and see that the LORD is good," says Psalm 34:8.

But How?

To live the life you truly desire, you must start immersing your thoughts in Scripture. But what if it isn't part of your life to regularly read, study and memorize the Bible?

Rather than give you the mechanics of digging into Scripture, I want to show you what immersing yourself in

Scripture is ultimately about. Techniques for Bible memory and Bible reading plans do exist, and we talk about them in several places throughout this book and in other First Place curriculum; but right now I want to point you to a Person, not a technique. That person is the Lord Jesus Christ. He is what reading Scripture is all about. When reading the Bible gives clarity to our minds, we will begin to live uncluttered lives. Reading Scripture is about knowing the God who will change our lives for His purposes and for our good. When we know more about Him, reading Scripture seems less like something we have to do and more like something we want to do. That can make all the difference in creating a sustainable habit that's truly good for us.

I want to suggest two ways that you can come to know the Lord. As you know Him, all of life begins to fall into place and make sense, including your thoughts that may have become cluttered by an unfiltered culture.

1. Our Job Is to Come

God's way is for us to willingly come to Him. We have a friend in Christ. Christ understands us and knows what we're going through. Are you weary from carrying a heavy burden today? God says, "Come to Me." Do you desperately need a friend who will listen and not judge? God says, "Come to Me." Do you need emotional healing from the ravages of life? God says, "Come to Me." Do you want to lose weight or have your health restored? God says, "Come to Me."

Only as we learn to come to God will we receive the help we so desperately need. When we come to Him, we will receive the power to stop the destructive behaviors we detest. When we come to Him, we will start feeling differently; anger will subside, fear will diminish and hope will return.

When we open the Bible, we find a real Friend.

2. It Doesn't Matter How We Feel

The beautiful part of immersing ourselves in Scripture is that we don't have to feel like it to do so. Coming to God is an act of our will, not our feelings; we choose to come to God. No person can make us open our Bibles and read, including the Lord. He created us with the ability to make a conscious decision to come to Him; our job is to do it.

How is that a beautiful thing? In Matthew 11:28, Jesus says, "Come to me, all you who are weary and burdened, and I will give you rest." When we open Scripture, good things happen. As we come to know Christ, we find that He is gentle and humble in heart, and we find rest for our souls. The Bible promises that His yoke is easy and His burden is light (see vv. 29-30).

Initially, we may not feel like coming to the Lord, but when we do so as an act of our will, we find a God who meets us exactly where we are. And that's beautiful.

The Promise: Just As We Are

God's way is for us to come to Him just as we are. He wants us to come when things are going great and when things are rotten. When we have messed up royally, God still loves us. We can come to Him early in the morning, late at night, while driving in traffic. All we have to do is show up and He is already there, waiting to meet with us.

There are many reasons why we don't come to God. It may be that even though we have accepted Christ as Savior and Lord, and we know in our minds that He has forgiven all our sins, we still feel dirty. God forgave us, but we can't forgive ourselves. We mistakenly believe that we can come to God only after we get everything cleaned up.

But until we come to God, our situation will only get worse. As we come to God, He will remove our guilt and shame and replace it with His love and acceptance. Staying away from Him will only make these feelings intensify. Come to God if you are full of guilt and shame. Hebrews 4:16 tells us, "Let us then approach the throne of grace with confidence, so that we may receive mercy and find grace to help us in our time of need."

Many of us fear God because we don't really know Him. Yet we can't know Him until we start coming to Him. When the word "fear" is used in the Bible, it often means reverence and awe. To fear God means that we recognize how great and mighty He is and we come to Him knowing that He is God and that we are not.

We may also fear God because we don't yet love Him deeply. God's way is the way of gentleness and kindness. One of my favorite memory verses is Isaiah 41:13: "For I am the LORD, your God, who takes hold of your right hand and says to you, Do not fear; I will help you."

I have been a Christian for over 50 years, and I can honestly say that there have been many times when I deserved severe punishment from God. In fact, I am so glad that I am not God, because I would surely have killed me by now! The amazing thing is that even in those times when God must correct me, He has never been harsh or unloving. How can I be afraid of One who loves me perfectly and only wants what is best for me?

In my darkest hours when I have chosen to come to God, He has rushed to meet me right where I am with open arms of love. I wish I could say that after all these years I never sin, but that would be a lie. I still do things that I hate and I don't do things that I desire to do. But when I come to God, He assures me that He loves me and that He's going to help me change.

The culture around you can be used for good and evil. If you do not filter what you see, hear or read, the negative side of our culture will clog your mind and lead you to destruction.

But there is a better way. When you dig deeply into Scripture, you will find a God who loves you and cares for you. By knowing

Him, you are able to discern your surroundings and make correct and healthy choices each day.

Won't you come to Him right now?

CHAPTER 10

Stop Controlling; Start Empowering

Trying to dictate what happens in our world only wears us out. Only when we allow people to make choices and live with the consequences are we on the road to health.

Though you grind a fool in a mortar, grinding him like grain with a pestle, you will not remove his folly from him.

PROVERBS 27:22

I was a bit startled one evening to see one of our neighbors and his 21-year-old son standing outside our front door. He and his son had just had a disagreement and asked if I would mediate.

The son, a landscaper, hired his dad to build a brick patio around a swimming pool for a client. At one point during the job, the dad left the site to go get supplies. While he was gone, his crew began to goof off, which prompted the owner of the house to phone the son to complain.

The dad wanted his son to remedy the situation in a specific way, but the son disagreed with his dad's method. The son wanted to run his business the way he saw fit.

I listened to the dad, who was doing all the talking. He's a good guy, but he's also the type of father who wants to control whatever situation he's in with anger. I could tell he wanted me to take his side. The son just had an exasperated look on his face. Both of them were obviously frustrated with each other.

I don't remember exactly what I said, but I think it was something about how my opinion didn't mean much, but I was sure they would work it out between them. I shared my opinion that although both of them had hurt feelings, ultimately the dad would have to let his son grow up. The dad responded, "You're right, even if that's not what I wanted to hear."

This was a prime example of a father wanting to control his adult child. Kids have to be able to grow up and make decisions—including mistakes—for themselves. The son was a man now; he was trying to run a business and work independently. But he would never learn what he needed to do if his dad was always hovering over his shoulder. The dad needed to stop trying to control his son and start letting him be.

In Control

What a waste of time and energy it is when we try to control the people and situations around us, particularly when we try to change those who don't want to be changed! A truth that most of us fail to realize is that we're powerless to change others. In whimsical fashion, Proverbs tells it like it is: "Though you grind a fool in a mortar, grinding him like grain with a pestle, you will not remove his folly from him" (27:22).

Whenever we try to manipulate a situation the way we want it to be, as opposed to seeing something for how it really is, we're exercising power where we shouldn't. When we try to control others, when we try to direct and dictate their lives, we are trying to create something that was never meant to be. It's emotionally exhausting to do this. Sometimes we just have to let people make choices and live with the consequences.

We can use a variety of methods to try to control other people and situations. Guilt, anger, bribery (presents), silence, disapproval—these can all be tools of control. Have you ever seen, heard of, or experienced some of the following situations?

- A husband promises his wife a new wardrobe only if she loses weight
- A boss keeps silent even when his workers do a good job
- A teenager is lazy and disobedient, but his parents still pay for his car, insurance, gasoline, clothes, food and entertainment
- A friend thinks she's responsible for her other friends' spirituality. If they don't go to church, it's all her fault. She thinks she hasn't prayed for them or witnessed to them enough.

When we try to control others, we wear ourselves out. When we try to order our world in ways that it was never meant to be, we become frustrated and discouraged. When we use our time, energy and effort in a futile attempt to control others, we're not using our God-given resources to do what He asks us to do—to practice self-control. Self-control, in this case, means that we let others be. We do not interfere in people's choices and the consequences of those choices.

We also tend to obsess about the people or situations we try to control. Obsession about other people and how we can change them drains our energy, clutters our mind and erodes our focus on God. And it undermines His will for our lives. The Lord invites us to abide in Him and to call on His power to bring about positive change in our lives. When we dwell on people, places and things that we're powerless to change, we don't have the time, energy or desire to live a life pleasing to God. In a vain attempt to control others, we find that we, too, are out of control.

The result is frustration, fatigue, anger, ulcers, burnout and more. Trying to control others hurts us and it hurts others by preventing them from learning, growing and changing for the better.

We all know that a more positive way exists. We can see a better way to live. It's found in a simple phrase.

STOP IT!

Just STOP IT!!!

STOP IT and STOP IT and STOP IT again.

In this case, we must stop controlling others and start letting people and situations exist as they are.

Letting It Be

No matter how hard we work to produce change in others, our efforts will always be in vain. Changing others is not our job, it's the Lord's. As a matter of fact, our best effort to change others often enables them to keep doing the very things we're trying to change! People have to make their own decisions. They must have the ability to choose the pathways they want in life and then deal with the consequences. Sometimes this means pain for them. And though it's hard for us to believe this is good, we have to let people exist in a painful situation if that's the choice they have made.

You see, like it or not, pain is God's messenger heralding the need to do things differently. People do not change until the pain of changing becomes less than the pain of not changing. When our efforts to control others keep them from feeling the natural God-given consequences of their actions, our helping becomes counterproductive.

Drs. Henry Cloud and John Townsend, in their book *Boundaries*, recall a story that illustrates the principle of trying to control others.

The parents of a 25-year-old man (we'll call the parents John and Jane Doe) came to one of the doctors with a request that psychologists hear a lot: They wanted the doctor to "fix" their son, Bill. When asked where Bill was, John and Jane answered, "Oh, he didn't want to come. He doesn't think he has a problem."

It seems these desperate folks had a long history of problems that began when Bill was very young. What had begun as minor problems while he was in school had now escalated. In recent years Bill had gotten into drugs, dropped out of college and was unable to hold a job. It was easy to see how much this couple loved their son, and they were heartbroken over the way he was living his life. It seemed that John and Jane had tried everything they knew to get him to change and live a responsible life, but all had failed. He was still using drugs, avoiding responsibility and keeping questionable company.

The Does had always given Bill everything he needed. They had made sure he had plenty of money while he was in college, because they had wanted Bill to be able to study and socialize rather than go to school and work a part-time job at the same time. When Bill flunked out of one college, John and Jane quickly arranged for him to go to another. When Bill crashed a car due to negligence, they bought him another one. The story of Bill's irresponsibility went on and on.

Finally the counselor stopped them and said, "I think your son is right. He doesn't have a problem."

"Did I hear you correctly?" asked the dad. "You don't think he has a problem?"

"That's right," replied the psychologist. "Bill doesn't have a single problem. You have them all for him. Bill can do whatever he wants. You pay, you fret, you worry, you plan, you exert energy—all to keep him going. He doesn't have any problems because you have taken them from him. All those things you told me about should be his problems; but as it now stands, they are yours."

The counselor's next statement surprised John and Jane even more: "Would you like me to help you give Bill some problems?"

John and Jane just looked shocked, but they asked the doctor to continue.

"Look at it this way," the doctor said. "It's like your son is your neighbor who never bothers to water his lawn. He doesn't have to, because whenever you turn on *your* sprinkler system, the water falls on *his* lawn instead. Your grass is turning brown and dying, but Bill's grass is green and lush. That is how your son's life is. He doesn't study, plan or work, yet he has a nice place to live, plenty of money and all the rights of a family member who is doing his part. As it stands now, he is irresponsible and happy, and you are responsible and miserable. We need to move the problems out of your yard and into his, where they belong. We need to give him a problem—one he has chosen to make for himself."[1]

Watering the Right Yard

Were you able to see yourself somewhere in that story? Is there someone in your life who is irresponsible and happy while you are responsible and miserable? Ask yourself this question: Has all my helping in this situation truly helped, or has it actually harmed me while shielding him (her) from the consequences God is trying to use to get him (her) to change? JUST STOP IT! Quit using your time and energy and financial resources to water someone else's lawn, especially when to do so leaves your own yard barren and brown.

Scripture shows us a better way in the parable of the prodigal son (see Luke 15:11-20). As the story begins, we see the son demanding his inheritance, even though his father is still alive. In Jewish society, that request was the same thing as wishing the father was dead. But the father doesn't react to the insult. He doesn't try to control his son. He could have lectured the son on all he had done for his son or reminded him of how a good son *should* act.

Instead, he let him be. The wise father simply divided up his fortune, gave his demanding son what was due him (*after* the father's death!) and watched him leave. When the son left, the father did not run after him, plead with him or promise him rewards for staying at home. He just let him go.

Did the father miss his son? Of course. We are told that he looked down the road daily to see if that might be the day his son would come to his senses and return home. But the father did not go after him. The wise father knew that dire consequences bring prodigal sons and daughters to their senses faster than any words ever spoken.

The tough love continued. When times were hard and the son was doing without, the father did not send him a care package. Did the father know what was going on in his son's life? Of course he did! But even though the lad had squandered his inheritance and was doing without, the father did not intervene. He did not send messengers to try to persuade his young son to come back home. Nor did the father use his power and influence to manipulate circumstances. He simply let his beloved son reap the consequences of his folly—all the way to living with pigs and eating swill. And when the son finally came to his senses, he came home to a loving father who was patiently waiting for his son's return.

Who do you identify with most? John and Jane Doe, who were desperately miserable about their son's irresponsible ways but enabled him to stay on that path? Or the loving father of the prodigal son, who knew that God-given consequences teach misbehaving sons and daughters faster than anything else?

Let Reality Be Reality

Our desire to control situations and people can affect so many areas of our life. Any time we don't let reality be reality, we are trying to control it. Trying to control will only frustrate and wear us out.

So what do we need to do? Start letting things exist as they truly are. We are not called to be anyone's savior, parachute, or get-out-of-jail-free card. We are called to love people, pray for them, offer them grace, provide education, if applicable, so they can make their own choices—and let them be.

What might life look like when you stop controlling others and simply let them be? It may look ugly for a time. It may look messy. People may become angry with you, because they have gotten used to being bailed out by you. They may even think you don't care. But the truth is, you do care. You care a lot. But letting others be is the most loving thing you can do. It's the type of tough love that is not afraid to do whatever is necessary, even when the necessary thing is hard.

Letting others be might look something like the following:

- Your son goes to school once in a while without clean socks. You've told him the only way he gets clean clothes is to put his dirty ones in the hamper. Because he didn't do that, he needs to deal with the consequences.
- Your best friend is jealous when you spend time with other friends. When you refuse to make excuses or apologize, she will be forced to deal with the consequences of trying to control and manipulate your friendship.
- Your spouse gets diabetes because of being overweight. This is so hard to let be, but nagging won't lead anybody to health.

I admit that I haven't always chosen the right path when it comes to letting people be, particularly when my own children were growing up. Sometimes there's a fine line between guiding our children, which is healthy, and making choices for them when the healthy thing to do is let them make those choices for themselves. I remember one time when my decision to let my daughter Shari have her own way proved to be a good time of growth for her. (Thankfully, the issue was not a serious one, so the consequences were not too painful.)

Shari was 15 and planning to go on a two-week summer trip to England with her youth choir. As a teenager, Shari was really into clothes. In her mind, going on a two-week trip meant she needed to bring two or three changes of clothes per day—at least.

There was only one problem: Each student was allowed to bring only one suitcase on the trip. It was a space issue for the airplane. And everyone had to carry their luggage wherever they went. One suitcase?! How was Shari ever going to manage?

Shari borrowed the biggest suitcase I had ever seen from my mom. It was a huge soft-sided, navy-colored monstrosity. She just kept packing and packing, cramming clothes in as tight as they would go. When the suitcase was finally closed, the sides were bulging. That suitcase must have weighed as much as a steamer trunk.

I knew that Shari would have a hard time carrying it. I mentioned that fact to her a few times, but I didn't forbid her from taking the suitcase crammed with clothes. I let her decision be her decision.

The very first call we received once Shari arrived in England told me that she had learned her lesson.

"Why didn't I listen to you?" she said. "I'm staying in a third-floor flat and had to carry it all the way to the top. This thing is so heavy—how am I ever going to lug this around for two weeks?"

I just smiled.

If this chapter has resonated in your heart, know that you

can stop controlling others and situations and start letting them exist as they are. You can either travel the path that leads to harm and destruction or the path that leads to health and healing. The choice is yours. With God's help, you will succeed.

Note

1. Henry Cloud and John Townsend, *Boundaries* (Grand Rapids, MI: Zondervan Publishing House, 1992), pp. 27-28.

PART 4:

—STRENGTH—

As we look at the fourfold composite of our lives—
heart, soul, mind and strength—"strength" is the word
used to describe the physical nature of our lives.
Our strength comes from our bodies and what we do
with our bodies—how we feed, care, nurture, exercise
and strengthen ourselves.

Bodies are incredibly important. Through our bodies we
carry out the daily acts of life. Our bodies are the tool the
Lord gives us to accomplish His plan here on Earth. By
creating sustainable healthy habits for our bodies, we can
live as the Lord intended us to live.

That's what the next three chapters will discuss.

CHAPTER 11

Stop Relapsing; Start Resisting

Once we get going on the right path, it's easy
to fall back into harmful habits.
We must make plans to guard our life.

Submit yourselves, then, to God. Resist the devil,
and he will flee from you.
JAMES 4:7

When my husband, Johnny, needed to have surgery to have a stint removed, I was surprised by how short the procedure was—only about 30 minutes. He was up and around by noon that day. It's funny, but when anything throws a curve into your life, even when it isn't serious, your whole world takes a hit. If you're not careful, the hit can shove you off track.

Johnny does a fair bit of cooking in our family, and he cooks a healthy cuisine. He'll cook up a pot of red beans with corn bread—no fat, but still tasty. Or he'll make linguini and meatless red sauce topped with steamed broccoli and carrots—absolutely yummy. When he had the stint removed, and although he was up and walking around, he didn't feel like cooking that night. Thankfully, he still had his appetite, so we went out for some Mexican food. The next day, Friday, we felt the same way. So we went out again—this time for seafood. Saturday we did the same thing. Sunday came and went, and we found ourselves eating in another restaurant. Four days of eating out in a row. The trigger was all because of Johnny's 30-minute surgery.

Eating out that much was not bad for us, because we still made good choices, but it wasn't as good as it could have been. When you eat out, you never know exactly how much fat, salt, sugar and preservatives are hidden in food. Plus, it's also a lot harder to set boundaries on portion control. You usually eat more than you would at home.

There were also temptations in the restaurants that we wouldn't encounter at home. At one point during our four-day excursion, Johnny ordered onion rings. These are okay for Johnny to have every now and then, but they are definitely a no-no for me. Sure enough, there they sat right in front of Johnny, and I had two of them. Two onion rings will not destroy my life, but they have the power to get me off track. Knowing my tendencies, it could have led me to eat the whole plate. The next day I would crave cheesecake. And so on and so on and so on.

The principles of this book are much easier to say than they are to put into practice—mainly because STOP IT! is not just a one-time event. It's a way of life. Even when we've said STOP IT! to a destructive habit, relapsing can be easy to do if we're not on guard, particularly against the small hits in life.

Stopping destructive habits requires planning and taking action. Paul tells us that the kingdom of God is not a matter of talk but of power (see 1 Cor. 4:20). Most of us who are trying to change destructive habits are very good at talking the talk and could probably write a diet book by ourselves. But it's not about lack of knowledge; we fail because we do not apply what we know. When it comes to STOP IT! it's easy to say the words. Walking the walk is more difficult.

Relapsing Is Easy

Have you ever noticed consistent patterns when you fall? Same time, same place, same companions, same circumstances, over and over again. We do want to submit ourselves to God and be obedient children, but we continue to stumble. We do not lack desire or motivation, but we don't heed the second part of James's admonition in James 4:7—we do not resist the devil. We fail to realize that friendship with the world is enmity with God (see Jas. 4:4). We're not successful in our quest to STOP IT! because we're not willing to eliminate the places, the circumstances and the relationships with people that lead us back into our disease. We're not successful in our efforts to STOP IT! because we're not willing to cut off the enemy's supply route! We're not willing to starve sin because we're not willing to eliminate the things that allow sin to flourish.

Elizabeth Crews, one of the First Place Networking Leaders in southern California, works as an addictions counselor with folks who often have a relapse problem. They quickly grasp the principles of recovery, excel within an inpatient treatment program setting and are often a role model to fellow patients. But then for some seemingly unknown reason, they lapse back into old habit patterns at a predictable time in their treatment program.

Elizabeth tells me that this usually happens when the exterior boundaries of the treatment center are removed and the person needs to use inner boundaries to resist temptation. In working with these patients, she has learned to quite accurately predict when the relapse will occur. No matter how high their motivation, some people fail to resist the devil by eliminating the people, places and things that will lead them back into old ways.

You and I are not immune to this kind of relapse. Going back to our destructive habits causes heartache, loneliness, disease and sorrow. All the same, it's easy to fall back.

There is a solution. A remedy exists to crush the destructive patterns of our lives and create sustainable, positive habits in our lives. These new habits can open up a life we never dreamed possible—a life filled with meaning, health and purpose. This life is well within our grasp.

But we've got to do something first.

A Sustainable Lifestyle

What's the solution?

STOP IT!

Just STOP IT!

STOP IT and STOP IT and STOP IT again.

In this case, we must stop relapsing and start resisting. We need to build into our lives a plan that guards us even when small triggers emerge that have the potential to knock us off track.

I believe that people relapse for three reasons: (1) We want what we want when we want it; (2) we fail to plan; (3) we fail to identify the one food that always gets us going in the wrong direction. By reversing these reasons, we can gain an understanding of how to stop going back to destructive patterns of choice.

Changing Our Pattern

Temptation can creep in so innocently. Often it appears harmless at first. It could be as innocent as two onion rings sitting on a plate in front of you that lead to a more dangerous pattern of temptation.

Hebrews 12:1 talks about how sin can easily entangle us. That's why we can trace a relapse pattern back to the same people, places, times and circumstances that create our unavoidable temptation and subsequent fall. When relapse happens, we have stopped walking on the path of fulfilling God's purpose for our lives. If you or I are going to STOP IT! we need to eliminate the things that allow sin to flourish in our lives. We must learn to cut off the enemy's supply route and starve sin. We need to purposely create circumstances that guard us from relapse.

What might such a plan look like? Here are a few suggestions.

- Take a different route on the way home from work—the one that doesn't lead by the ice cream store.
- Enlist a friend to become an exercise partner. (We aren't as prone to slack off when we're accountable to someone.)
- Purchase an online tracking system that sends a report of our website visits to someone we trust.
- Cut up all credit cards to stay away from unrestrained spending.
- Have an "escape route" to handle our emotions. (If we feel our anger rising toward our kids, we need to have a step-by-step action plan for what we will say and do and where we will go.)

Incidentally, this is one of the reasons I encourage people to join a First Place group in their area. On a weekly basis, First Place meetings help educate people to make healthy choices for themselves. We have built-in accountability for support and encouragement, and we offer numerous resources to help people create a healthy, sustainable lifestyle. (See the contact page for First Place at the back of the book.)

We Want What We Want When We Want It

"Self-indulgent" is a word we don't hear a lot today, but it basically means that we want what we want when we want it.

Typically, and sadly, we're actually encouraged to be this way by a lot of today's advertisements and marketing strategies.

The Bible offers a different path: "Do not think about how to gratify the desires of the sinful nature" (Rom. 13:14). One of the fruit of the Spirit is self-control. When we exercise self-control, we don't always get what we want—not immediately anyway. Peter also calls us to be "clear minded and self-controlled so that [we] can pray" (1 Pet. 4:7). As long as we are continually thinking about ways to make ourselves feel better in an instant-gratification type of way, we will not abstain from the things that wage war against our souls (see 1 Pet. 2:11).

One of the worst examples of temptation to self-indulge that I can think of is a buffet restaurant. Why do we go to these places? Who thought up "all you can eat"? It's a bad situation for people who struggle with weight loss. First of all, we think we need to get our money's worth—so there's no way we're just going to plunk down $12.95, eat a salad and leave. Second, there is absolutely no portion control built into the buffet system. You just load up your plate, chow down, then head back for more while your dirty plate is whisked away. You can eat several plate-fuls before anyone notices.

I think of all-you-can-eat buffets as troughs. Glance around at folks who frequent these restaurants. Many are overweight. And look at the food piled high on their plates. All-you-can-eat buffets are a recipe for disaster.

My coworkers and I sometimes go to a cafeteria for lunch called Luby's. We like it because it's quick and we can get what we want of the right kind of food in the right portions. It has become a game to see how little we can spend for lunch. I can get a spinach salad, fresh fruit, vegetable and a roll for $3.99. It's healthy and quick, and I have accountability because I'm not eating alone.

All of us need to build into our lives patterns that do not allow us to be self-indulgent.

We Fail to Plan

Soldiers, police officers, lifeguards and pilots practice over and over again how they will act in crisis moments so that they will revert to this default knowledge when they are faced with a real crisis. If you and I are going to be successful in our attempts to STOP IT! we must learn to do the same.

We must plan and then mentally and sometimes physically rehearse how we are going to handle stressful situations. In the words of the old adage, we must plan our work and work our plan. For those of us who are trying to stop destructive eating habits, that means planning meals and having healthy food available. It means eating according to a preplanned schedule so that we never get too hungry. And it means eliminating everything that would keep us from planning our work and working our plan.

We Fail to Identify the Most Problematic Food

What is the one food (and you know what that food is) that always gets you going in the wrong direction? It might be a particular creamy food like ice cream or cheesecake (that's my thing!). It might be salty, crunchy food such as chips or snack crackers. Most of us can be quite successful at losing weight until we give in to the one food that just happens to be our "drug" of choice. Once we start eating this particular food, we seem to quickly get off track.

For some people, their problem food might be something as simple as peanut butter. Although peanut butter is a good food (it contains monounsaturated fat), it is high in calories. If peanut butter causes you to relapse and you find yourself eating it by the spoonful, then you might need to stay away from it until you reach your weight goal. Kay Smith, of First Place, says that it was always a piece of cheese for her. She would have a healthy breakfast and a healthy lunch. But in the late afternoon she wanted a snack and would go to the refrigerator to slice off a piece of cheese. This was something she could have but was also a food that started her on a binge of eating other foods that she couldn't have and still lose weight.

Creating Your Plan Today

Think about a consistent pattern that leads you to destructive lifestyle habits. Perhaps it's a group of friends who have become eating buddies, and unless you're enjoying a lavish meal, you can't enjoy one another's company. Maybe it's a family member (or members) who are threatened (perhaps unconsciously) by your success and who unwittingly sabotage your plans to change. Maybe it's a favorite restaurant that serves the bread pudding with blueberry sauce you just can't resist. Maybe it's being in the kitchen alone late at night, or it's the fat- and sugar-laden snacks you continue to put in your cupboard "for the children" (or grandchildren). Maybe it's driving past your favorite store on the way home and finding that your car goes on autopilot into the parking lot!

Make a list right now of ways you can guard against relapse and start resisting. Take a few moments to fill in the blanks below or on a separate piece of paper. You may want to work through this section with an accountability partner.

My problem area is: _____

When I tend to relapse I'm
    with the following people _____
    at the following location _____
    at the following time(s) _____
    usually feeling _____

because the following has happened in my life

_____.

You may need to make more than one list. Do you see a pattern emerging yet?

Let's keep going.

My goal is to not fall into the habit of _____

_____

because I know it creates the following harmful circumstances:

_____.

I want to create a new sustainable habit. Therefore I will guard myself by changing the following circumstances: _____

_____

removing the following temptations: _____

_____

staying away from the following places, at these times, with these people: _____

_____.

Remember, you are not keeping this record to condemn yourself but to become aware of Satan's schemes to keep you in a failure mode when it comes to what you really want to accomplish. Recognize that with every commitment comes temptation, and that Satan will consistently use what he knows from experience works on you! Don't be ignorant of the people, the places and the things he uses to pull you back into his web. We must resist those things that wage war against our souls. We've got to STOP IT! by starving sin.

What Is the One Thing?

When it comes to creating a sustainable, healthy lifestyle, we must draw near to God. Jesus calls us to abide in Him. He says, "Apart from me you can do nothing" (John 15:5). But in order to draw near to God, we must resist the devil. Remember James's words at the beginning of this chapter? Friendship with the world is enmity with God. Until we are willing to abstain (another word for STOP IT!) from the things that wage war with our souls, we will not enjoy fellowship with the Father.

Are you familiar with the story of the rich young ruler in Mark 10:21? "One thing you lack," Jesus said to him. "Go, sell everything you have and give to the poor . . . Then come, follow me."

We often think that Jesus' words mean that we have to sell everything before we can follow Christ. But I think Jesus was getting at something different here, because elsewhere he meets other rich people and doesn't say the same thing. I think Jesus was telling the rich young ruler to identify the one thing that kept him from wholeheartedly following Christ and then eliminate it from his life. For the ruler, it was possessions.

Each of us must ask ourselves the same question. We need to have the courage to rid our lives of whatever it is that is holding us back. What I must give up may not be the same for you. Yet the question is the same. We all must ask ourselves, What is the one thing that keeps me from following the Lord wholeheartedly? What is the one thing that keeps me from living the way the Lord intended?

Which path will you choose today? Are you willing to eliminate what leads you back into your destructive ways? Are you willing to starve sin so that you can enjoy the banquet God has prepared for you? Are you prepared to create the plan that guards your life and leads you to success?

Jesus stands at the door knocking. If you open the door, He will come in and dine with you and, in His presence, you will have a continual feast.

CHAPTER 12

Stop Retreating; Start Running

Stopping a destructive habit and replacing it
with a healthy one is the first big step.
But we can't leave it at that.
Sustaining the new habit is all-important if
we truly want to succeed.

Let us run with perseverance the race marked out for us.

HEBREWS 12:1

I am a runner.

Well, not really, not anymore. I work out with weights and I
walk on a treadmill every morning at 6:00 A.M., but I don't actually sprint barefoot down the beach at Galveston like some scene
out of *Chariots of Fire*. At age 63, I'm afraid my knees can't handle
that type of running anymore.

But still, I am a runner. I run with perseverance the race
marked out for me.

You have a calling to be a runner too.

Running is a figure of speech used many times in the Bible.
Psalm 119:32 instructs us to "run in the path of [God's] commands." Paul describes his ministry in Philippians 2:16 as running. First Corinthians 9:24 tells us to "run in such a way as to
get the prize."

Think of running as the good journey of your life. When you run, you create a purposeful, sustainable, balanced lifestyle that has a God-honoring goal in mind. Your goal is the prize that Paul talks about in 1 Corinthians 9:24—the prize that comes when you run well and finish strong. What is the prize? There is more than one. There's the heavenly prize that comes when you put your faith in Christ. But there are also earthly prizes along the way—benefits of the healthy decisions you make as you live in the grace of Jesus Christ and sustain the good habits that promote health.

The prize may look different for each of us. I approach my race as someone who has spent too much time walking and crawling in life. One of the ways I run today is by having accountability built into virtually every area of my life. What are some specific ways that I am accountable? (I mention these only to give you some examples to help you identify your own way to run.)

- I teach a weekly First Place class that keeps me studying the Bible regularly. If I'm not prepared, then I don't have anything to teach. So the good pressure of teaching keeps me studying Scripture.
- I exercise with my good friend Pat each morning. Pat and I also use this time as we walk side by side on treadmills to say Scripture verses to each other. We have about 120 verses memorized at this point in time. It takes just 3 minutes to say 10 verses.
- When I go out to lunch, I go with friends who are committed to health in the same way that I am.
- I keep in contact at least once a month with one of my mentors, Joy Stephens. Joy is a pastor's wife and has been a dear friend for over 35 years. Joy was my Sunday School teacher when our kids were little and was a godly influence in my life. She gave me Scriptures

> to memorize and called me every Saturday evening to
> see if we were going to church the next morning. She
> was the one who first told me I needed to teach others.

How about you? What ways do you run your race? It may be that reading this book is your first step. But it takes a plan of action, too. You have to be purposeful about deciding to run or else you have taken the first step back in retreat.

The Stranded Sailors' Problem

A woman once told me that she used to walk three miles a day. Then she caught a cold—something minor—and she didn't walk for a entire year after that.

Now that's retreating, and it's so easy to go that direction. We are never called to stop the race. We're called to create a sustainable lifestyle that honors the Lord. Once we stop a destructive habit, we must replace it with a healthy habit and focus on sustaining the good.

The writer to the Hebrews tells us to throw off everything that hinders us. That includes those old habits and patterns that keep us mired in the muck. We need to untangle and throw off the things that keep us entangled so that we can run the race marked out for us. That's the STOPPING concept we've been talking about all the way through this book. To ensure that we are successful in our efforts, Hebrews goes on to tell us how to accomplish that feat: Fix your eyes on Jesus, the One who came to show us how to live a life pleasing to God (see Heb. 12:2)! That's the STARTING point.

Do you remember the story about the Russian mini-sub that was stuck on the ocean floor? The sub was entangled in a web of fishing line and cables that prevented it from coming to the surface. Inside the sub was a crew of seven men. Their oxygen supply was low, but they were powerless to sever the cords that kept them fastened to the ocean floor.

They were not without hope, however. Their distress signal, which was received by the Russian navy, was immediately sent to the Russian government who sent out an international call for help. British and American crews rushed to the scene.

The sailors on board the sub were given specific instructions. They were to lie down, conserve energy and oxygen, shut down any unnecessary equipment and wait expectantly for hope to arrive.

So many times our lives look like that scene inside the mini-sub. How much like that mini-sub our lives must at times look to God. It's easy to get ourselves in danger and have our resources run low. That's when the temptation comes to retreat back to our old habits.

The problem is, we don't act like those stranded sailors. What do we fail to do?

- *We do not send out a distress signal.* When temptation comes to us, we may think that we can get back on track by ourselves. Or, we may be too ashamed to ask for help or think we'll bother someone if we do ask. But we must enlist people who care for us in order to run our race.
- *We do not stop doing the things that drain our energy and resources.* Our lives are not limitless, and we cannot do everything. One of the sure-fire ways to sink into old habits is to take on too much—even good activities can push us off track and cause us to retreat into old habits. We need to find out what God has called us to do and then do it—and do nothing else. Even good things may not be *best* for us if they cause us to be unable to do the better things we're called to do.

For example, I absolutely love national Bible teacher Beth Moore. Every Tuesday night at our church there is a Bible study class that uses curriculum written by her. Not only that, but since Beth is a member of our church, she actually teaches this study herself. I'd absolutely love to go to this study. But when I go to it, I don't get home until 10:00 P.M. or later. So I quietly say no to attending the study.

My specific calling right now is to three things: to the directorship of First Place, to my husband and to my family. The only way I can succeed at this threefold calling is to begin my mornings early. I can't do this if I get home late at night. So I must say no to something, even if it's good, in order to devote my time and energy to my calling.

- *We do not obey God's clear commandments.* God's instructions are found throughout Scripture. As we immerse ourselves in His Word and yield ourselves to the power of the Holy Spirit, God's pathway becomes clear to us. Often, the answer to our problem is staring us in the face but we choose not to obey God's voice. When we find ourselves in danger, it is often because we have not followed God's clear commandments.
- *We do not wait in expectant hope, confident that help is on the way.* The key to waiting is prayer. If we are struggling with the temptation to quit our race, we must enlist the power of the Lord. God has a plan for us, and His help arrives in His perfect time. Sometimes His timing doesn't look like our timing. Are you in danger of retreating? Then pray! Pray right now! Don't go looking in the garbage can of old habits for a solution. Look to the Lord.

Retreat from your race will never bring about the life you hope it will. Retreat only brings the destruction that bad habits produce. Bad habits are what cause us to feel overburdened, joyless, lonely, bad tempered and in poor health.

A new life is well within our grasp. In *The Message*, Eugene Peterson describes this life in Galatians 5, which I have paraphrased: What happens when we live God's way? He brings gifts into our lives, much the same way that fruit appears in an orchard—things like affection for others, exuberance about life, serenity.

What is the solution that will help you stop retreating and start running?

It's found in one phrase. STOP IT!

Just STOP IT!

STOP IT and STOP IT and STOP IT again.

You must stop the destruction and replace those negative habits with new behaviors that promote life, health and well-being. Then you must learn to sustain those new behaviors and not retreat back into old ways. You must stop retreating in order to run the good race.

New habits do not sustain themselves. The Christian life is a continual "weed and feed" process in which we *keep saying no* to the bad and *keep saying yes* to the good.

I hope that by now in the course of reading this book, you have made some commitments. Here are some possibilities for change:

Instead of remaining sedentary, you have begun to exercise.

Instead of worrying, you have started praying more.

Instead of eating junk food, you have filled your cabinets with healthy food.

Instead of repressing feelings, you have begun to open up to trusted friends.

Instead of going out with your eating buddies, you have begun to make new friends who support your new, healthy lifestyle.

The question now is, How do you continue on this path?

I want to suggest three ways that you can continue on the good course set out before you. Think of these as ways to run and to keep running, and to not retreat.

Run by Committing to Self-Discipline

When we begin to run, often one of the first emotions we must deal with is the feeling of deprivation. Something that was important to us—our old habit—is no longer there. When we feel deprived, a battle begins. Suddenly, the things that we can't have take on a life of their own. Cookies call from the cupboard. Ice cream screams from the freezer. Candy jumps right out of the dish. Whatever our forbidden fruit is becomes our preoccupation.

That's when the evil one seizes the opportunity to convince us that God is withholding something good that we deserve. From the beginning, Satan has used feelings of deprivation as part of his arsenal of deception when tempting God's children to go outside the boundaries God has established for their welfare.

The wisdom of Proverbs 15:32 tells us the truth: "He who ignores discipline despises himself." Self-discipline is not deprivation. Self-discipline is actually a hallmark of self-care. It is a lack of discipline that is true deprivation. We despise ourselves when we ignore the God-given limits and boundaries that protect our health and well-being.

Once our old habit is no longer there, the true feeling that can replace it is humility. Humility comes when we no longer insist on living life our way but follow the Lord's plan instead. In humility there is great trust. God says that He will give us the desires of our hearts. By stopping something that hurts us, we open the door to something better that He can give us.

Run by Looking Forward

Saint Augustine once said that God longs to fill our hands with good things, but we are so busy grasping the things of this world that we can't receive His gifts. Not only does that comment speak to the goodness of God as the Giver of every good and perfect gift, but it also contains another valuable truth.

In order to take hold of our new life, we must let go of our past. We cannot cling to one and grab hold of the other. It is impossible to reach backward and forward at the same time. As long as we dwell on our destructive habits, our mistakes and regrets, we will not be able to focus on the new habits God wants to bring to our lives. To receive, we must let go.

Run by Taking Action

My friend Elizabeth Crews coined a great phrase: *Someday Isle*. Someday Isle is where many people, unfortunately, live. It's the land of good intentions. People who live there dream about a better tomorrow but fail to take and keep taking the action steps that would make their dreams become reality.

How easy it is to say, "Someday I'll begin to exercise" or "Someday I'll quit eating food in secret" or "Someday I'll be consistent about Bible study and prayer." Let me tell you a secret—tomorrow is always tomorrow. Tomorrow never comes. For dreams to be reality, that "someday" must be today.

Let's take a step right now to sail away from Someday Isle.

Stop for a moment and think about the destructive habit(s) that so easily entangles you. Find a piece of paper and write it down. What destructive behavior do you need to replace with life-affirming action? If you record a list of behaviors, apply the triage principle. Select the destructive behavior that is the most life threatening and work to STOP that behavior first. For example, if you are still smoking cigarettes and spending too much time playing computer games, which one is more injurious to your health?

Once you've identified the most serious problem, find one or two Scripture verses that directly address that negative behavior. Write those verses on 3x5-inch index cards. The next time you find yourself tempted to do the thing that keeps you entangled, say STOP IT! out loud if necessary. Then read (or recite from memory) the truth of God's Word—and keep repeating it until the compulsion leaves you. Resist the devil and submit yourself to God. If you don't have your Scripture cards with you, say STOP IT! and then begin singing the words of a favorite praise song. Nothing makes the devil flee faster than to hear us praising God!

Run to Win

One of our First Place leaders, Mark Gutierrez, is a great example of someone who runs well. Mark runs spiritually, but he also runs physically. Recently, he ran a half-marathon—13.1 miles. This is amazing, considering that Mark used to be (as he describes himself) "a 300-pound couch potato who couldn't even walk around the block."

Mark joined First Place seven years ago. He's under 200 pounds now. Last year at a leadership summit, when personal trainer Beverly Henson issued a challenge to everybody there to join her in running a full marathon a year from then, Mark signed up.

He hadn't run in a long time. But he started slowly, first by training to run a 5K. It was the very first race he'd ever been in, but he knew if he was going to prepare for a marathon, he needed to prepare on a smaller scale first. He set a goal of 30 minutes and completed the 3.1-mile course in 30 minutes and 1 second.

The following week he began training for a half marathon. He decided on a goal to complete the run in 2 hours and 20 minutes. To help him keep the goal in mind he recited Galatians 2:20 at all 13 of the 1-mile markers.

Mark described the half-marathon in an e-mail:

By mile 6, I was feeling like I might not finish. But I persevered and kept going. I was actually ahead of my time until I hit the 10-mile marker. I was tired, really tired. Then just before hitting mile 12, the course started going uphill. At one point almost everyone was walking. My time kept slipping and I was afraid I wasn't going to be able to keep going. It appeared as if the end of that hill was nowhere in sight.

Finally, about three-quarters of a mile before the end, the ground leveled off. I gave it all I had and crossed the finish line with an official time of 2 hours 21 minutes and 14 seconds. Just 74 seconds slower than my goal, but I finished those 13.1 miles!

Mark is well on his way to his goal of completing a full marathon. I know he'll make it, because he's learned how to sustain his new health habits.

You can do this, too. Not all of us are called to run actual marathons, but all of us are invited on some sort of good race ahead. Once you have begun to run, the resources are within your grasp to keep you on course. You don't have to retreat. You can press on to the prize!

Stop Deviating; Start Tracking

Make a plan and stick to it. It's that simple.

Make level paths for your feet and take only ways that are firm.

PROVERBS 4:26

When it comes to maintaining a healthy lifestyle, one of my biggest temptations springs up when I hang out with my grandkids.

I have eight grandkids that I love so much, and I love to be with them! They're all so great—Cara, Carl, Christen, Katherine, Tal, Amanda, Hunter and Harper. Our family celebrates all birthdays and holidays together. But the thing about grandkids is that it's so easy to deviate from the plan when they're around. When I'm around them I tend to think, "Oh, I'm going to hurt somebody's feelings if we don't eat some birthday cake" or "No one will notice if I just eat this cupcake."

Little deviations can add up quickly. The challenge is to let the fun keep happening with my grandkids without getting knocked off track. And that's the part that's up to me.

Tamara Fisher, a First Place Leader in Rockwall, Texas, has learned the secret that allowed her to stop the damaging effects of self-destructive behavior. Tamara lost 140 pounds by following the First Place program. How was she able to be so successful? Tamara shared her recipe for success at a recent leadership summit.

"I just stuck to the plan," Tamara declared. "No matter what else was happening, I stuck to the plan. I didn't deviate for birthdays, holidays, vacations or celebrations. I just stuck to the plan."

Isn't it amazing how God can provide such a simple solution to our complex problems? All we need to do is stick to the plan—to continue on pathways that are firm. Success is found in the process, and the process means sticking to the plan no matter what.

Small Animal, Big Problem

We live in a society in which it is easy for our actions to be governed by circumstances rather than inner convictions. We see this happen in all areas of life: marriage, relationships, finances and the way we care for God's temple, our physical bodies.

Instead of following God's plan and taking only pathways that are firm, we are tempted to make up our own rules. Instead of heeding God's call to holiness (to be whole and complete human beings who reflect His purpose and plan), we are tempted to make choices based on changing circumstances. Instead of just sticking to the plan, we deviate from the plan and then wonder why we don't reach our goals and dreams.

Song of Songs 2:15 describes a small animal that can create a big problem: "Catch for us the foxes, the little foxes that ruin the vineyards, our vineyards that are in bloom."

Catching the little foxes is an important concept for anyone who wants to stop destructive habits and start beneficial ones. When most of us contemplate evil, we conjure up visions of fierce predators that pose imminent danger to our security. But the devil will not send a growling grizzly bear when a cute little fox will serve the same purpose.

That's why Solomon, in his wisdom, tells us to catch the little foxes that nibble away at the tender vines, destroying the crop-producing blossoms before they can develop. The little foxes are the small areas of distraction in our lives that keep us from focusing on the one important thing. Little foxes seem harmless enough—a birthday party here, an office function there. But little foxes can turn out to be insidious predators that chew and trample until they've destroyed our good progress. Then our destructive habits are once again in full swing. What started out small is now eroding our peace and serenity. We feel distracted and frustrated. We're headed down the wrong path once again—the one that keeps us feeling miserable.

The next time you're being chewed by a little fox, practice the method we talked about a while back—playing the tape all the way through. Remember the word we used—"trajectory." Trajectory is the curve an object takes as it leaves one location and heads toward another—like a tennis ball when it is lobbed over a net. Trajectory is about how the choices we make today—even the small choices—affect what happens to us in the future. Ask yourself, What is the trajectory—the end result—if I deviate from my plan even a little bit?

Can you picture where that trajectory might lead?

There is a solution to an off-course trajectory.

It's found in one phrase. STOP IT!

Just STOP IT!

STOP IT and STOP IT and STOP IT again!

Stop deviating from the plan and start sticking to the plan. The little areas that seem so inconsequential are really nothing of the sort. When the goal is health—in all areas of life—we need to be fully committed to that end.

Getting Our Bodies in Order

Perhaps the best way to apply STOP IT! to the physical realm is to picture the stop signs that are part of our driving routine. Each time we come to a stop sign, we are commanded to come to a full and complete stop, to look both ways, to remember the rules of safe driving and proceed when it is safe to do so.

Can you picture it? When you come to a stop sign, don't think of saying, "It's my birthday, I'll just sail on by today" or "I just got a terrific raise, so I don't need to drive on the right side of the road today!" If you based your obedience to the rules of the road on the changing circumstances of your life, you would never reach your destination. Yet you are doing the same thing when you deviate from your weight-loss plan because of birthdays, raises, anniversaries, office parties, church potlucks and the like.

I can't say this more gently. The hard fact is this: Good health takes work. Period. Good health will not happen automatically. It will not happen if all we do is hope for it. It means saying no to the little foxes and putting down the doughnut. It means walking around the block, making good choices, stopping harmful behaviors and starting healthy ones. Good health will not happen any other way.

We who are Christians can often hang ourselves out to dry in this area, so I want to spend some time discussing the importance of committing to a physical plan and not deviating from it once we're on it. Sometimes we think we're above the rules of nature. God is a supernatural God, so physical laws don't really apply to us, do they?

This kind of thinking is a huge mistake. There is danger in thinking that if we can only become "religious" enough, we will become healthy automatically. Do you know what I mean by that? We think that if we just pray enough or read enough Scripture or attend enough seminars or do enough good works, our physical maladies will be magically transformed. People caught in this trap say things such as:

- I don't need to exercise; my body's not really that important anyway. God is much more concerned about my soul.
- Here I am at a church potluck. I can't refuse to eat any of Jane's apple crumb cake—that would hurt her feelings. I'm doing a good thing here, so deviating from my weight-loss plan won't matter just this once.
- If I just pray hard enough, I know I can overcome the temptation to look at pornography. I don't need to put any safeguards on my computer. I don't need to set up any accountability. The only action I need to take is to pray.
- My husband is so abusive, I just don't know how I can handle it anymore. But I shouldn't say anything. I definitely shouldn't leave—good wives never do that. I'm sure God will bless me if I just keep my eyes on Him.

Prayer, fellowship and keeping our eyes on Christ are of utmost importance, but Scripture shows us that if we're going to achieve wholeness, we must take steps in that direction. God is ultimately the One who transforms us, yet He calls us to actively participate in the process. Changing our lives takes our will as well as the power of the Holy Spirit.

In this case, we must pay specific attention to our physical recovery. We can't ignore our bodies. God can heal people miraculously if He chooses to do so, but He usually chooses to work in natural ways. That means we need to take action in the area of having a healthy body.

Two examples come to mind. The first is found in Romans 12:1-2: "Therefore, I urge you, brothers, in view of God's mercy, to offer your bodies as living sacrifices, holy and pleasing to God. . . . Do not conform any longer to the pattern of this world, but be transformed by the renewing of your mind. Then you will be able to test and approve what God's will is—his good, pleasing and perfect will."

This verse is a call to offer our bodies as living sacrifices. It's also a guide to preparing ourselves to live for Him. Let's summarize the three aspects of being a living sacrifice as outlined by Paul.

- *First—offer your body as a sacrifice pleasing to God.* This means that you give your complete being to the Lord. Simply and directly you say, "God, my body is Yours," and you actively take steps toward physical restoration. For instance, you might deliberately put down the remote, get up off the couch and go outside for a walk as an act of your devotion to the Lord. Offering your body to the Lord means that you make a plan for healthy living and stick to it.
- *Second—renew your mind.* This is the obedience step where you commit your attitudes, thoughts, feelings and actions to the Lord. As your mind is continually being made new by the spiritual input of God's Word, by prayer and through Christian fellowship, your life will continually be transformed. This means that you deliberately set aside the mindless book or magazine you're reading and pick up your Bible. We are to immerse our thoughts in truth.
- *Third—discern God's good, pleasing and perfect will.* As you commit your body to Him and are transformed in your mind, you become more like Christ. Then you are able to discover what pleases the Lord.

Interestingly, secular addiction treatments follows Paul's template even though Christians sometimes do not. What we see in addiction treatments is this:

- *Physical recovery*—first abstain from a substance or process. Get off the bottle, stop overeating or get out of a house where abuse is happening. First set the boundary on the physical substance or process.
- *Mental transformation*—learn how to think clear thoughts once your brain is no longer under the influence of a "drug of choice."
- *Spiritual awakening*—begin to connect to God, to your inner self and to others.

The second illustration is found in 1 Peter 4:7, in which Peter tells us to "be clear minded and self-controlled so that [we] can pray." Note that physical sobriety (being clear minded and self-controlled) also comes first in this verse. I'm not suggesting that people under the influence of overeating cannot pray. There are plenty of stories in which people turn to the Lord in the midst of addiction, such as when a drunk accepts the Lord while he's on Skid Row. But if we are believers and we are addicted to something, we can't ignore the fact that the Bible tells us our spiritual growth is hampered unless we first focus on the health of our bodies.

Start with your body. Does that sound strange to you? We seldom hear that message in a sermon or seminar. But the order in both Romans 12:1-2 and 1 Peter 4:7 starts with the body. *Offer your body* to God. *Be sober minded* so that you can pray. We can't ignore the physical. If we're caught in an addiction, we begin the restoration process by pulling the plug on our destructive habit.

This physical recovery is sometimes called detox. That may sound like a harsh term when talking about overeating, but it simply means that we clear our body of the toxic affects of a drug. We can detox from any number of addictions—food, shopping, gambling, extreme risk-taking, pornography—anything that has us under its spell. Even though we are not ingesting a substance that makes us drunk, the chemical reaction to the addictive rush is making us not think clearly. And that's still being drunk.

An addicted person (someone who is still practicing a harmful behavior) seldom has the ability to think clear thoughts. Alcoholics Anonymous refers to thoughts under the influence as "stinkin' thinkin'." We also see this same disordered thinking in any addiction. Until the damaging substance or process is removed, we cannot begin to acquire the mind of Christ. A mind under the influence continues to conform to the things of the world.

Once the body has gone through detox and the brain begins to sober up, we can begin to renew and transform our minds with the Word of God. Can you begin to see the futility of those who think that if they just read enough Scripture or go to enough seminars or read enough self-help books they will be magically fixed? We cannot begin to renew an intoxicated mind. We have to stop putting the harmful substance in our mind that makes it intoxicated in the first place. That's why folks in health programs such as First Place who do the spiritual commitments but not the physical commitments seldom make progress. Until the body is sober, the mind can't absorb the truth. Finally, after the body is sober and our thoughts are clear, we can begin to discern God's will and connect on a spiritual level with God, with self and with others.

So we see recovery occurring this way: the physical leads to the mental, which leads to the spiritual.

Interestingly, relapse occurs just the opposite way: We slip spiritually (lose our connection to God) and then begin to think disordered thoughts that lead to a physical relapse.

Perhaps this is more information that you need, but I want you to better understand why I just can't stress enough that physical recovery is so important. We just flat out cannot achieve lasting success until we are "sober minded and alert," as Scripture says. And that takes physical sobriety.

I will say it once again: Health takes work! We cannot ignore our physical recovery. Once we make a plan, we have to stick to it. Period. Our decisions have serious consequences if we don't. We're not playing a game when it comes to our physical health. The hard, cold facts are that some of you will soon be gravely ill or even dead if you don't change your habits. Too many people want the parts of a plan that are easy for them (and that make them feel good), but they don't want to do the tough STOP IT! work that requires physical action. But you can't have one without the other.

Please stop your destructive behavior today and start your road to health.

Help Is Here

The good news when it comes to physical restoration is that we are not alone in this battle. We have the power of the Holy Spirit. Our new way of thinking and acting involves two key components. The first is our will. We have to firmly decide to take a plan of action and then do it and not deviate from the plan. Second, we are able to depend on the life-changing power of the Holy Spirit in our lives. God is ultimately the One who creates lasting good change in our hearts and lives. God changes us, yet we play a role too. We've got to want to change, we've got to take steps in that direction, and we've got to keep taking steps in that direction. With God's help, you can make those changes.

It seems strange that our bodies come first in this process. But that's often where a person has to start when it comes to total life change. Once our bodies are fully committed to the Lord and free from the toxins of our addictions, our thoughts will clear and we will be able to see a new view of the glory of God.

CHAPTER 14

Staying Stopped; Staying Started

Final thoughts for the road ahead.

Stand firm and hold to the teachings we passed on to you,
whether by word of mouth or by letter.
2 THESSALONIANS 2:15

Have you ever wished that you could
    stop thinking certain thoughts,
    stop acting a particular way,
    stop returning again and again to bad habits
        so that you could be a different person than you are now?

You can do it!

You have the tools. You can stop that destructive habit today and start a positive habit to replace it that will help facilitate health and healing in your life. It won't always be easy. It will take your will and determination, but with the Lord's help, your life will change.

I want to offer a few last thoughts about your life from this point on. If you're like me, resolve and determination are easy to muster at the start of a project. But somewhere about 10 days to 2 weeks into a new plan, the initial commitment begins to wane.

Maybe this isn't the right program for me after all, you think. *This is much harder than I thought it would be,* you say to yourself on a sigh. *The timing just isn't right. I'll do it after the holidays, after my birthday, after vacation, after the kids are back in school.* It's easy to revert back to the comfort zone that is the cause of our discomfort.

How can we make this a life-long plan? How do we stay stopped on the path of destruction and stay started on the road to sustained health?

There is hope.

Remember the Three

Whenever Elizabeth Crews talks to a group of newly recovering alcoholics and drug addicts, she takes a handout with her with three short slogans typed across the page in large, bold print. Each person in the group is asked to take a handout, put it in their recovery notebook and repeat these three simple sayings to themselves several times each day:

My recovery is my top priority.

No matter how bad my circumstances might be,
I can always make them worse by returning to my old behavior.

I can stand this time of change.

Take a moment to write those three sayings in your journal or notebook before you finish reading this book. They are important truths to remember for anyone desiring to stop the downward spiral of destructive behavior.

What do these three simple sayings have to do with stopping destructive behavior? Everything! For most of us, stopping is not the problem; staying stopped is the continual challenge and the point at which we all too often fail.

Often, the real reason our resolve wanes has nothing to do with the program, the difficulty of the task at hand or the timing of our endeavors. The reason we *stop* stopping is because we have failed to factor in one very important recovery concept: the discomfort of withdrawal—that period between stopping the old behavior and having new coping tools in place that support the new, healthy lifestyle to which we aspire. An anonymous writer put it well: "Between the bondage of Egypt and the glory of the Promised Land, we must all go through the desert." In the desert, our courage fails unless we are prepared to encounter the discomfort that is sure to surface. The desert experience called withdrawal is where uncomfortable things can dwell.

There is an old saying in addiction treatments: If you want to know why you do something, don't try to figure out why; just stop the behavior and you'll quickly learn why! If you've just stopped a habit, right now you may be asking yourself why you stopped. Life may be very hard right now. And I want you to know that is okay. Life will get easier—and better. Right now, the discomfort of stopping a destructive habit is simply part of the narrow path you are called to travel.

For those of us who have stuffed our emotions for many years, the primitive emotions that begin to bubble to the surface when we stop our out-of-control emotional eating can be frightening. Emotions such as anger, fear, guilt, shame, humiliation, unworthiness, loneliness, sadness, grief and despair emerge. Those of us who suffer from out-of-control eating learned at a very young age to elevate our sagging spirits and deal with all those unacceptable emotions we were not allowed to express by stuffing them down with food. Years later, the very behavior that was once essential to our survival has become self-defeating and destructive. If we're going to stop the behavior, we have to learn to deal with the emotions that will begin to surface once they are no longer buried beneath the excess food we have used to keep them under control.

I have a friend who remembers such a time. It occurred during her second week after stopping a destructive eating habit and starting a positive eating habit as outlined in the First Place Live-It Plan. It was about 4:00 P.M. one afternoon and she was preparing dinner—a difficult time for any of us who are trying to abstain from eating between meals. Her grandsons were visiting, and they were squabbling while the TV was blaring, the phone ringing and the dog barking. My friend's coping ability had worn so thin that it was almost nonexistent.

Suddenly she found herself thinking, *I can't stand this one more second!* That's when she spied the box of sugary cereal on the kitchen counter. Immediately she convinced herself that she had two choices, and only two choices: either she could take her building frustration out on her grandsons or she could stuff those awful feelings down with handfuls of cereal.

In that decisive moment, the cereal won. Minutes later she held an empty box in her hand and wondered what had gone wrong. Her initial resolve had been so strong, her intentions so God-honoring; but somehow she had failed to stand firm in her commitment.

Why?

In that critical moment, my friend tells me now that her recovery had not been her top priority. She managed to make a bad situation worse by reverting to her old behavior. Also, in her initial enthusiasm and determination to stop her self-destructive eating, she had failed one essential ingredient—to come up with a plan to handle the uncomfortable feelings that would begin to surface when she stopped stuffing them down with food. She had neglected to factor in the discomfort of withdrawal. As a result, she reverted back to her old coping behavior.

When Emotions Come Up

What we must realize is that our decision to STOP IT is more than a one-time decision. STOP IT is an ongoing process. One of the side effects of this—the side effect that can so easily knock us off track—is that stopping it can bring us face-to-face with all those emotions we have worked so hard to hold inside, usually in our futile attempts to please people.

The truth is, those supposedly negative feelings we don't allow ourselves to feel are natural human emotions that need to be expressed in healthy, life-affirming ways. Fear. Anger. Frustration. Loneliness. None of these emotions is wrong in and of itself. God gave us the full spectrum of emotions. Jesus experienced all of these, except perhaps for fear. He was angry with people who desecrated His father's house. He was often frustrated with His disciples. He grew lonely and tired. He wept at Lazarus's grave.

Emotions are not wrong. Emotions can be expressed in healthy ways. But having that knowledge and being able to apply it to our circumstances are two different things. That's why our most valiant efforts at lasting weight loss can fail. Sometimes, we just have to go back to the basics and start from there.

My recovery is my top priority.

No matter how bad my circumstances might be,
I can always make them worse by returning to my old behavior.

I can stand this time of change.

Putting those principles into practice takes planning, because without a plan, it is very easy to fall back into our old destructive habits. If we are ever going to stand firm in our commitments to change, we are going to have to learn a better way to deal with the ups and downs of life.

Here's one simple plan. Before you go to bed each night, write down some thoughts about the next day. It could be as simple as:

What I will eat . . .

When I will exercise . . .

What positive actions I will take to cope with the stress of daily life without my faithful but destructive coping mechanism . . .

Rather than reaching for the sugar-coated cereal, we learn to take a walk or stop what we're doing and play with the grandkids rather than sitting them in front of the TV while we hurry to complete the tasks at hand. Instead of trying to be perfect, we learn to strive for excellence by putting our recovery before serving meals on time or juggling a schedule that leaves no time to take care of ourselves. Rather than stuff our emotions, we learn to express them in healthy ways such as exercise, journaling, crying out to God, and opening up to trusted friends. As we do these things, we find that we can stop turning to food for comfort, solace and relief.

If putting our recovery first means we need to stop what we're doing at the moment and journal or read Scripture or pray or call a friend, then that's what we need to do. Does that mean we neglect other responsibilities? No. But the priority has shifted. Now that our inner reserves are no longer used to hold down unwanted emotions, we have more energy than before and more patience with those who need our time, attention and direction. We know at a heart level that reverting back to our old coping behavior will only make our situation worse. Most of all, we learn that with God's help we can stand it! By His grace, and His grace alone, we learn to positively deal with the emotions that we have stuffed for years.

One last practical suggestion: There is another word for "STOP" that I would like to share with you—"HALT." By using the letters in that word, you have an acrostic that becomes another important "stop it" guideline.

Never allow yourself to become too

Hungry,

Angry,

Lonely or

Tired,

because the moment those things happen, your ability to stop it is in jeopardy.

Help in Time of Need

I want you to take away everything else for a moment and just listen to what is strongest on my heart.

If I could say anything to you, it would be this: *You can do it.* The healthier, more purposeful, more joyful life you imagine is within your grasp.

But the only way you'll do it is with a strength that's not your own. The pathway of health absolutely does take our will power. But real, lasting change will not come about unless we rely on the Lord Jesus Christ. We must commit our ways to the Lord and ask for His help. Yes, He has a wonderful plan for our lives. But we must ask Him to help us implement that plan.

When you don't want to exercise—ask God for help.

When you don't feel like memorizing Scripture—ask God for help.

When you feel tempted to overeat—ask God for help.

When the pressure to slide back into that destructive habit tempts you—ask God for help.

He comes alongside us when we are obedient. First Corinthians 10:13 offers a wonderful promise: "No temptation has seized you except what is common to man. And God is faithful; he will not let you be tempted beyond what you can bear. But when you are tempted, he will also provide a way out so that you can stand up under it."

It is my prayer that this book will help you make both the one-time decision and the ongoing commitment to stop doing the things that keep you in defeat and despair, and start doing and keep doing the things that lead to a better life.

God is with us. He will strengthen us and keep us from harm as we learn to trust in His goodness and grace and face the wild beasts that keep us in bondage to out-of-control behavior. By His grace, and His grace alone, we can stand firm, and STOP IT!

Don't Miss the Companion Bible Study to *Stop It!*

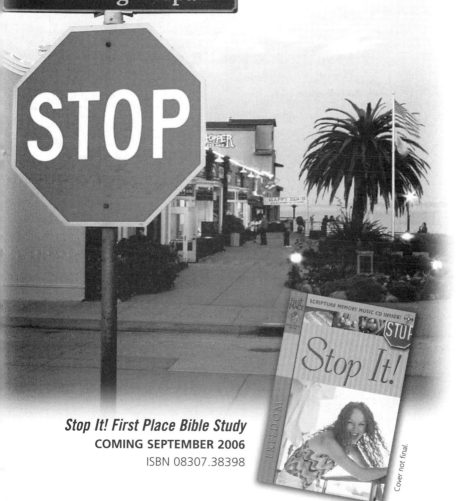

Stop It! First Place Bible Study
COMING SEPTEMBER 2006
ISBN 08307.38398

Cover not final.

THE BIBLE-BASED WEIGHT-LOSS PROGRAM USED SUCCESSFULLY BY OVER A HALF MILLION PEOPLE!

Are you one of the millions of disheartened dieters who've tried one fad diet after another without success? If so, your search for a successful diet is over! But First Place does much more than help you take off weight and keep it off. This Bible-based program will transform your life in every way—physically, mentally, spiritually and emotionally. Now's the time to join!

ESSENTIAL FIRST PLACE PROGRAM MATERIALS

Group Leaders Need:

■ **Group Starter Kit** • *ISBN 08307.33698*

This kit has everything group leaders need to help others change their lives forever by giving Christ first place!

Kit includes:

- *Leader's Guide*
- *Member's Guide*
- *First Place* by Carole Lewis with Terry Whalin
- *Giving Christ First Place* Bible Study with Scripture Memory Music CD
- *Introduction to First Place and Nine Commitments* DVD
- *Orientation and Food Exchange Plan* DVD
- *Leadership Training* DVD
- myfirstplace.org three-month trial subscription
- One package of 25 *First Place* Brochures

Group Members Need:

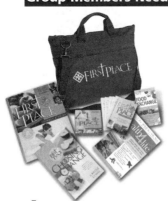

■ **Member's Kit** • *ISBN 08307.33701*

All the material is easy to understand and spells out principles members can easily apply in their daily lives.

Kit includes:

- *Member's Guide* • *Choosing to Change* by Carole Lewis
- *Motivational CDs* • *Food Exchange Pocket Guide*
- *Commitment Records* • *Health 4 Life*
- Scripture Memory Verses

Available at bookstores everywhere or by calling 1-800-4-GOSPEL. **Join the First Place community and order products at www.firstplace.org.**

Gospel Light

Bible Studies to Help You Put Christ First

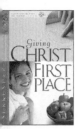

Giving Christ First Place
Bible Study
ISBN 08307.28643

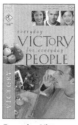

Everyday Victory for Everyday People
Bible Study
ISBN 08307.28651

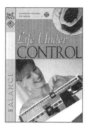

Life Under Control
Bible Study
ISBN 08307.29305

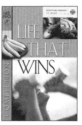

Life That Wins
Bible Study
ISBN 08307.29240

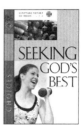

Seeking God's Best
Bible Study
ISBN 08307.29259

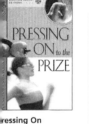

Pressing On to the Prize
Bible Study
ISBN 08307.29267

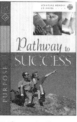

Pathway to Success
Bible Study
ISBN 08307.29275

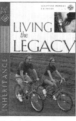

Living the Legacy
Bible Study
ISBN 08307.29283

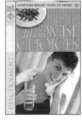

Making Wise Choices
Bible Study
ISBN 08307.30010

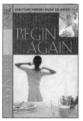

Begin Again
Bible Study
ISBN 08307.32330

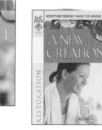

Living in Grace
Bible Study
ISBN 08307.32349

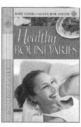

A New Creation
Bible Study
ISBN 08307.33566

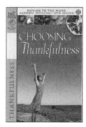

Healthy Boundaries
Bible Study
ISBN 08307.38002

Choosing Thankfulness
Bible Study
ISBN 08307.38185

Available at bookstores everywhere or by calling
1-800-4-GOSPEL. **Join the First Place community
and order products at www.firstplace.org.**

Gospel Light

Also from Carole Lewis

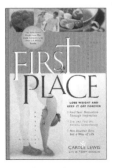

First Place
Lose Weight and
Keep It Off Forever
Carole Lewis with *Terry Whalin*
ISBN 08307.28635

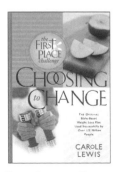

Choosing to Change
The Bible-Based Weight-Loss Plan
Used by Over a Half Million People
Carole Lewis
ISBN 08307.28627

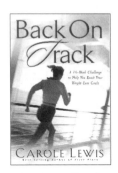

Back On Track
A 16-Week Challenge to Help You
Reach Your Weight-Loss Goals
Carole Lewis
ISBN 08307.32586

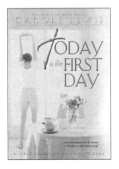

Today Is the First Day
Daily Encouragement on the
Journey to Weight Loss and a
Balanced Life
Carole Lewis, General Editor
ISBN 08307.30656

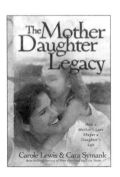

The Mother-Daughter Legacy
How a Mother's Love
Shapes a Daughter's Life
Carole Lewis and *Cara Symank*
ISBN 08307.33353

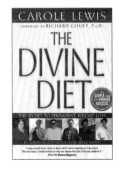

The Divine Diet
The Secret to Permanent
Weight Loss
Carole Lewis
ISBN 08307.36271

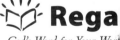